www.harcourt-inter

Bringing you products from all Ha... companies including Baillière Tindall, Churchill Livingstone, Mosby and W.B. Saunders

- ▶ **Browse** for latest information on new books, journals and electronic products

- ▶ **Search** for information on over 20 000 published titles with full product information including tables of contents and sample chapters

- ▶ **Keep up to date** with our extensive publishing programme in your field by registering with **eAlert** or requesting postal updates

- ▶ **Secure online ordering** with prompt delivery, as well as full contact details to order by phone, fax or post

- ▶ **News** of special features and promotions

If you are based in the following countries, please visit the country-specific site to receive full details of product availability and local ordering information

USA: www.harcourthealth.com

Canada: www.harcourtcanada.com

Australia: www.harcourt.com.au

Baillière Tindall   CHURCHILL LIVINGSTONE   Mosby   W.B. SAUNDERS

The Menopause and HRT

SECOND EDITION

Kathy Abernethy

Clinical Nurse Specialist
Menopause Clinical and Research Unit
Northwick Park Hospital
Harrow, Middlesex

With a contribution from

Denise Tiran

Principal Lecturer – Complementary Medicine/Midwifery
School of Health
University of Greenwich
London

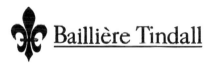 Baillière Tindall

EDINBURGH LONDON NEW YORK PHILADELPHIA ST LOUIS SYDNEY TORONTO 2002

BAILLIERE TINDALL
An imprint of Harcourt Publishers Limited

© Harcourt Publishers Limited 2002

✤ is a registered trademark of Harcourt Publishers Limited

The right of Kathy Abernethy to be identified as the author of this work has
been asserted in accordance with the Copyright, Designs and Patents Act 1988

First edition 1997
Second edition 2002

ISBN 0 7020 2635 2

British Library Cataloguing in Publication Data
A catalogue record for this book is available from the British Library

Library of Congress Cataloging in Publication Data
A catalog record for this book is available from the Library of Congress

Note
Medical knowledge is constantly changing. As new information becomes
available, changes in treatment, procedures, equipment and the use of drugs
become necessary. The author and the publishers have taken care to ensure
that the information given in this text is accurate and up to date. However,
readers are strongly advised to confirm that the information, especially with
regard to drug usage, complies with the latest legislation and standards of
practice.

The
publisher's
policy is to use
**paper manufactured
from sustainable forests**

Printed in China

Contents

Chapter 8 Non-hormonal Methods for Coping with Menopausal Symptoms 131

Denise Tiran; Introduction; The nurse and complementary and alternative therapies; An introduction to the most commonly used therapies; *Homeopathy*; *Bach flower remedies*; *Acupuncture and acupressure*; *Osteopathy and chiropractic*; *Herbal medicine*; *Aromatherapy*; *Reflexology*; *Massage*; *Nutritional therapy*; *Hypnotherapy*; *Yoga*; *Alexander technique*; Using complementary and alternative therapies for specific symptoms during the climacteric phase; *Anxiety, irritability and mood changes*; *Breast tenderness and discomfort*; *Headaches and migraines*; *Tiredness, lack of energy and insomnia*; *Hot flushes and sweating*; *Dysmenorrhoea and menorrhagia*; *Poor concentration and memory loss*; *Vaginal dryness*; *Mobility and prevention of osteoporosis*; Conclusion; References

Chapter 9 Patient Support 155

Decision-making; Sources of information; *Media*; *Primary healthcare team*; *Protocols*; *Providing information*; *Dedicated clinic*; *Audit*; *Community pharmacists*; Questions patients ask; Conclusion; References

Appendix: Resources 181

Index *187*

Foreword

I am delighted to have been asked to write the foreword for this much-awaited second edition of Kathy Abernethy's book, *The Menopause and HRT*. The first edition was a valuable and practical pocket-sized reference tool, and I am confident that this new edition will be equally successful. Although written primarily for nurses, all health professionals involved in the care of women will find it of great benefit in their work. It will also be of interest to the non-medical reader who is looking for some expert advice to help steer her through this stage of her life. It is easily read, well referenced and includes a useful 'questions and answers' section containing plenty of constructive advice.

The National Health Service continues to change rapidly, and our professional environment, whether hospital- or community-based, is very different from even a decade ago. Efforts to improve patient healthcare have resulted in frequent reforms of primary care teams and a flood of new guidelines. Clinical governance has assumed increasing importance in the professional workplace, and nurses, often the only point of regular patient contact, are now at the forefront of this change.

Nurses are frequently the linchpin in a multi-disciplinary team and can be a catalyst for progress. Their diverse training ensures they are the natural leaders in health promotion, outreach and patient advocacy, and they can move effortlessly between these roles. Their professional responsibilities and skills have steadily been extended, and the boundaries between nurses' and doctors' roles are becoming increasingly blurred. In primary care, appropriately trained nurses are already managing the total care of specific patient groups (e.g. those with asthma or diabetes and those requiring contraception). Nurses are also in an ideal position to advise women about the menopause and to supervise the management of their hormone replacement therapy (HRT).

As this book goes to press it seems likely that prescribing rights will soon be extended to more nurses and will cover a wider range of medicines. This will not only enhance patient care, by providing quicker and more efficient access to healthcare, but also make better use of nurses' skills and allow doctors more time to deal with complicated cases.

All health professionals have a responsibility to keep themselves regularly updated. Our knowledge of the menopause and HRT is continually being challenged by new research data, and the pharmaceutical companies offer a sometimes bewildering array of new products. Even those of us who are specialists in the field find it difficult to remain updated. Kathy Abernethy's book will be an invaluable reference book for us all.

The Menopause and HRT has been thoroughly revised and takes account of new research into the menopause and the ageing process. It explains new products and routes of delivery of HRT, and offers practical advice on giving a woman information about what to expect at this stage in her life, starting her on HRT and monitoring her progress. A fascinating new chapter, 'Non-hormonal methods for coping with menopausal symptoms', has been added for this second edition. This chapter has been written by Denise Tiran, an expert in complementary and alternative medicine, and clearly explains some of the alternative therapies currently available. Increasingly women ask for advice about alternatives to HRT, but it is an area in which few nurses have the relevant knowledge and expertise. Denise Tiran's chapter has been written from an evidence-based perspective and will enable us to give better advice.

As well as being updated to reflect the latest knowledge on HRT, there is a wealth of practical information that will enable health professionals to run an effective service for menopausal women. Written in an easy to use way, *The Menopause and HRT* is well referenced and has a 'resources' section which will be helpful for professionals and non-medical readers alike.

Every year that passes sees an increase in life expectancy, and more and more women will live half their adult lives in a post menopausal state. The challenge for all health professionals is to enable them to lead a healthy, active and fulfilling life right through to their old age. *The Menopause and HRT* represents an important resource in the achievement of this aim.

Gilly Andrews

Preface

The menopause has come of age! For much of society (although sadly, still not all), the menopause is now discussed freely by women both at places of work and in many social situations. Over the past 5–8 years, there has been a huge interest in the menopause by the media (sometimes distorted or inaccurate) and a rapid increase in the number of therapies available to women. Just look in any health food shop and observe the number of packets of pills aimed at 'midlife women' or women 'at the change'. Look in women's magazines and tabloid newspapers and see how the menopause is widely discussed and debated. But still we meet the stereotypes: menopause is assumed to happen at the age of 50 years, even though many women experience it much earlier – even in their twenties or thirties. The hot flush is assumed to be the worst symptom, yet for some women it will be the psychological symptoms that concern them most. Women hope that by 'living a healthy life' they will not encounter problems, but menopausal symptoms may affect even the healthiest of women, and sometimes factors outside her control will influence the health of a woman at the menopause and afterwards.

Women are beginning to understand that there is more to the so-called 'change of life' than simply the cessation of periods. Women want information about what happens to their bodies at the time of the menopause. They want to know what to expect in the way of symptoms and experiences. They want to know what they themselves can do or take to make it easier, and they want to know what measures are required to protect their long-term health. Many women want to take responsibility for their health and make their own decisions about whether or not to use medical interventions. They understand that health is more than 'the absence of disease' and want to invest time and effort into maintaining their physical, sexual, emotional and spiritual health.

So, where do women find out more? This book is written primarily for any health professional involved or interested in guiding women through the maze of issues relating to the menopause and its consequences. This may be a nurse working in primary care, those working in community health clinics, gynaecology nurses, or those working in specialist women's health clinics. Other health professionals, such as general practitioners or doctors working in the field of sexual health, should find something relevant to their practice. Students new to the area of women's health issues will find it an informative text and those regularly working in the field should find it an invaluable update.

The first edition of *The Menopause and HRT* was widely recognized as a practical handbook to the menopause. This edition has been completely updated, incorporating new evidence and practice in relation to the menopause and heart disease, osteoporosis and other medical conditions. The topic of early menopause is discussed, and in particular the unique needs of the women to whom this occurs. The section on hormone replacement therapy (HRT) has been updated to include new routes of delivery, new guidelines for management and evidence-based practice. Risks and side-effects are discussed comprehensively. New treatments such as selective (o)estrogen receptor modulators (SERMs), bisphophonates and phyto-oestrogens are described and discussed. The practical aspect of this book emphasizes the topics that women themselves ask about and helps you to address them comprehensively. The resource section has been developed to include useful websites as well as addresses.

A new chapter for this edition is Chapter 8 by Denise Tiran on 'Non-hormonal methods for coping with menopausal symptoms'. Many women do not want to use HRT, and many seek advice about therapies other than HRT. For those of us working in the field of menopause, this has meant trying to encompass a whole new area of expertise. This completely new, comprehensive section discusses complementary therapies from an evidence-based perspective, and is written by an expert in that field. Her contribution to the book is invaluable and will be of interest to all those who want to broaden the discussion beyond HRT and include complementary therapies in their discussions with women – a truly holistic approach.

The challenge to all of us working in the field of menopause is to counsel women and communicate with them in a way that enables them to be knowledgable about the choices and confident with their decisions. Only then will they truly enjoy the best of health at the menopause and beyond. If this book helps us to do that, then it has achieved its aim.

July 2001   Kathy Abernethy

Abbreviations

BMU	bone multicellular unit
BTB	breakthrough bleeding
CAM	complementary and alternative medicine
CHD	coronary heart disease
DoH	Department of Health
DXA	dual-energy X-ray absorptiometry
ERA	Estrogen Replacement and Atherosclerosis (Study)
FIM	Foundation for Integrated Medicine
FSH	follicle stimulating hormone
GI	gastrointestinal
GIFT	gamete intrafallopian transfer
HDL	high-density lipoprotein
HERS	Heart and Estrogen/Progestin Replacement Study
HIV	human immunodeficiency virus
HRT	hormone replacement therapy
IU	international units
IUS	intrauterine system
LDL	low-density lipoprotein
LH	luteinizing hormone
LHRH	luteinizing hormone releasing hormone
PMT	premenstrual tension
POP	progestogen-only pill
QCT	quantitative computed tomography
SERM	selective (o)estrogen receptor modulator
TCM	Traditional Chinese Medicine
TENS	transcutaneous electrical nerve stimulation
WHO	World Health Organization

1

What is the Menopause?

We have all heard and read about 'the menopause' but the term often means different things to different people. To some women it is simply an explanation of a physiological change taking place in their bodies. To others, the word itself triggers negative thoughts about middle age and loss of femininity. Most women will recognize that the time of the menopause is a time of hormonal disturbance, but many will not understand precisely what those changes are or what causes them to happen. This chapter will help you understand the hormonal influences that result in the menopause and therefore enable you to explain to your patients what is happening to their bodies. Later chapters will look in more depth at the consequences of these changes.

DEFINITIONS

Strictly speaking, the term **menopause** simply means *last menstrual bleed* and as such cannot be diagnosed until after the event.

The phase of time either side of this last bleed is described as the **climacteric** and it is during this time that many women experience physical and psychological symptoms, along with the emotional changes that some women will attribute to 'the menopause'.

In practice, both health professionals and women themselves use the term 'menopause' to include all aspects of this phase of life. Women talk about going 'through the menopause', referring to the months or even years of physical and emotional turmoil that may occur at this time.

A World Health Organization (WHO 1981) report on the menopause uses the following definitions:

◆ **Menopause**   Permanent cessation of menstruation resulting from the loss of ovarian follicular activity.
◆ **Perimenopause** (or climacteric)   The period immediately before the menopause with endocrinological, biological and clinical features of approaching menopause, and at least the first year after the menopause.
◆ **Postmenopause**   The era following the date of last menstrual bleed which cannot be determined until 12 months of spontaneous amenorrhoea has been observed. See Figure 1.1.

ONSET

In the UK, the majority of women experience the menopause at around the age of 51 years, although it commonly occurs as early as 45 years or as late as 56 years.

Menopause may occur at a very early age in some women, even in their twenties and thirties. This is described as a **premature**

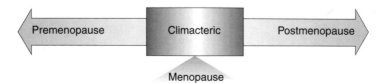

Figure 1.1 Phases of the climacteric.

menopause and such women deserve special attention, both in terms of physical care and also with regard to emotional support (see Ch. 4).

Studies have shown a relationship between mother's and daughter's menopausal age, suggesting that variation in menopausal age may be determined genetically (Cramer et al 1995, Torgeson et al 1997).

Age of menopause does not seem to be affected by:

◆ race
◆ use of oral contraception
◆ number of pregnancies
◆ age of menarche.

Smoking, however, does appear to bring forward the age of menopause by 1–2 years (McKinlay et al 1985, Sharara et al 1994).

WHAT HAPPENS AT THE TIME OF THE MENOPAUSE?

Hormonal influences

In order to understand how menopause occurs it is important to have a basic understanding of the normal female physiology during reproductive years.

During menstruation, low levels of oestrogen and progesterone are released into the bloodstream. The hypothalamus controls the secretions of these hormones through the release of luteinizing hormone releasing hormone (LHRH), which then stimulates the pituitary gland to produce follicle stimulating hormone (FSH). FSH, in turn, stimulates the ovaries (see Fig. 1.2) to produce oestradiol, which causes the endometrium to proliferate. As circulating levels of oestradiol increase, FSH and luteinizing hormone (LH) levels fall until around day 14 of the cycle. LH concentration then peaks and ovulation generally occurs (Fig. 1.3). If fertilization does not take place, oestrogen

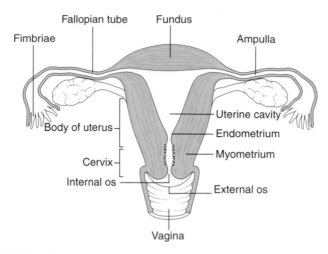

Figure 1.2 The female sexual organs.

and progesterone levels fall and the endometrium is shed – menstruation takes place. The falling levels of oestrogen and progesterone are detected by the hypothalamus and the cycle starts again.

From around the age of 35 years, the natural cycle becomes less predictable and ovulation may not occur in every cycle. Oestrogen levels fall and, as a result of the negative feedback system of the pituitary and hypothalamus glands, more and more FSH is released in an attempt to stimulate ovarian function. When oestrogen levels fall too low to stimulate endometrial growth, bleeding stops altogether and the menopause occurs.

Follicle stimulating hormone

Hormonal changes begin well before a woman sees an alteration in her menstrual pattern. Fluctuations in the levels of FSH and LH occur throughout the perimenopause, eventually peaking 2–3 years after periods stop and remaining high for the next 20 years or so, unless hormone replacement therapy (HRT) is taken (Teede & Burger 1998). FSH levels fluctuate widely during the menopausal transition.

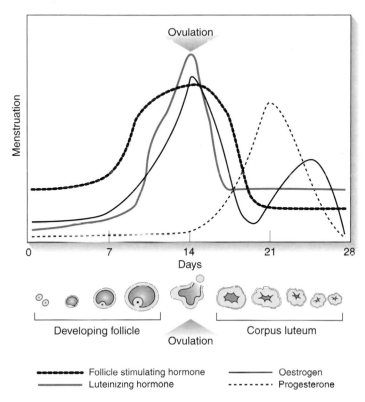

Figure 1.3 Normal menstrual cycle.

Oestradiol and oestrone

In the premenopausal woman, both oestradiol and oestrone are present, with oestradiol being the dominant hormone. Both are secreted by the ovaries but oestrone is also available through conversion in fatty tissue of the hormone androstenedione, which is secreted by the adrenal glands. Oestrone is biologically less active than oestradiol. After the menopause, the ratio of oestradiol to oestrone changes (Table 1.1), with oestrone becoming the dominant hormone. There may be transient periods of excess oestrogen, even with raised FSH levels (Teede & Burger 1998).

Table 1.1 Hormone changes following menopause

Hormone	Change in concentration
Oestradiol (E2)	↓
Oestrone (E1)	↓
Ratio of E2 : E1	Reverses
FSH	↑
LH	↑

↑, Increase; ↓, decrease

Measuring hormones

Many women believe that they need a blood test to confirm whether or not they are menopausal. In practice such tests are often unnecessary. Symptoms of the menopause do not correlate with actual levels of circulating oestrogen. Some women experience symptoms whilst maintaining relatively high oestrogen levels, whereas others, even with lower levels, may not have such bad symptoms.

Measurement of FSH levels will help diagnose the menopause, but as levels fluctuate widely in the perimenopause repeated determination of the level would be required to be certain of an accurate result. Measuring FSH or oestradiol concentration will not help in predicting whether or not a woman needs HRT. However, FSH levels may be useful in the following circumstances:

◆ hysterectomized women (see Ch. 4)
◆ diagnosis of premature menopause, which may have medical or psychological implications (see Ch. 4)
◆ to confirm lack of ovarian function for women seeking advice about contraception (see Ch. 5).

Effect of hysterectomy on menopause

It is possible that, even if the ovaries are conserved at the time of hysterectomy, vascular supply to the ovaries may be compromised, resulting in the menopause occurring earlier than it otherwise would (see Ch. 4; Siddle et al 1987). If a woman experiences an early menopause as a result of hysterectomy, but is asymptomatic, she could be at increased risk of osteoporosis and cardiovascular disease if that early menopause is not detected.

LIFE EXPECTANCY

Women approaching the menopause can now expect to live for many more years; many women are living into their eighties and beyond (Fig. 1.4). It is therefore becoming increasingly important to women that the postmenopausal years are as healthy as those before the menopause. Women often ask, 'Why must I think about the menopause, when my grandmother just got on with it?' The truth is that far fewer women of her grandmother's generation lived for many years after the menopause. It is not the menopause that has changed in character (although we do have a greater understanding of the physical changes now), but rather that women's expectation of life beyond the menopause has changed.

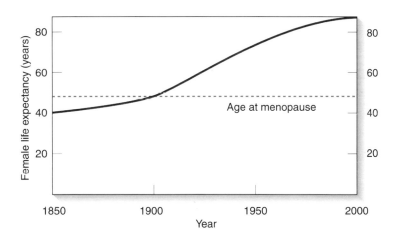

Figure 1.4 Changing life expectancy.

CONCLUSION

The menopause is a natural event which marks the end of fertility and the end of periods. The menopause itself is merely the outward manifestation of all the hormonal changes that will occur in a woman at this time. Helping women to understand the physiological causes of menopause and reminding them how their bodies normally function is the first step in helping them to come to terms with their changing body and then with all the other changes that may be occurring at the same time.

REFERENCES

Cramer DW, Xu H, Harlow BL (1995) Family history as a predictor of early menopause. *Fertil. Steril.* **64**: 740–745.

McKinlay SM, Bifano NL, McKinlay JB (1985) Smoking and age at menopause in women. *Ann. Intern. Med.* **103**: 350–356.

Sharara FI, Beatse SN, Leonard MR et al (1994) Cigarettes smoking accelerates the development of diminished ovarian reserve as evidenced by the clomiphene citrate challenge test. *Fertil. Steril.* **62**(2): 257–262.

Siddle N, Sarrel P, Whitehead MI (1987) The effect of hysterectomy on the age of ovarian failure: identification of a subgroup of women with premature loss of ovarian function. *Fertil. Steril.* **47**: 94.

Teede H, Burger HG (1998) The menopausal transition. In: Studd JW (ed.) *The Management of the Menopause, Annual Review*, pp. 1–12. Parthenon, London.

Torgeson DJ, Thomas RE, Rand DM (1997) Mother's and daughter's menopausal ages – is there a link? *Eur. J. Obstet. Gynecol. Reprod. Biol.* **74**: 63–66.

World Health Organization (1981) *Report of a WHO Scientific Group, Research on the Menopause.* Technical Report Series 670. WHO, Geneva.

2

Short- and Intermediate-term Symptoms

If the menopause simply represented an end to periods and to the possibility of having children, many women would accept it gratefully, even if those feelings were tinged with an element of sadness. An adjustment would be made to a new life era, and life would continue.

For some, the menopause is a relief, signifying the end of bleeds, the reliance on contraception and the monthly battle against premenstrual tension (PMT). For such women, the menopause is a positive experience. Relief is expressed particularly by women who have had problematic periods. Hunter & O'Dea (1997) describe many experiences of women during the menopause transition:

'I get hot at times, but it doesn't bother me. If it's hot, I just open a window...'

'You think hot flushes? – poof nothing... but you can actually feel the sweat tingling down your head when you wake at night, then you are tired all the next day...'

'It doesn't make me feel older, if that's what you mean.'

'I feel no different inside.'

'Once the menopause is over, it doesn't seem so very long to being old. It is a bit frightening...'

However, the menopause may bring with it agonies as well as blessings! Books and magazines would have women believe that menopausal women are in their 'prime of life', yet distressing symptoms and hormonal upheaval can make a woman feel anything but in her prime. The menopause is often called the 'change of life' and some women would say that it is a change for the worse: distressing symptoms, weak bladder and the beginning of the battle against the ageing process.

Of course, not everything that happens to a woman and her body during mid life can be blamed on the menopause. Hormones play a significant part in physical changes at this time, but some changes are similar in both men and women, and cannot be blamed solely on hormones. Other changes may arise as a direct consequence of a less than perfect lifestyle as the effects of smoking or dietary habits may become more obvious. This chapter outlines the symptoms that are commonly identified as being related to the climacteric, both physical and psychological. Long-term consequences of oestrogen deficiency are discussed elsewhere.

INCIDENCE

The list of potential menopausal symptoms appears endless (Fig. 2.1). Fortunately, no woman experiences all the symptoms and indeed some women experience no obvious symptoms at all.

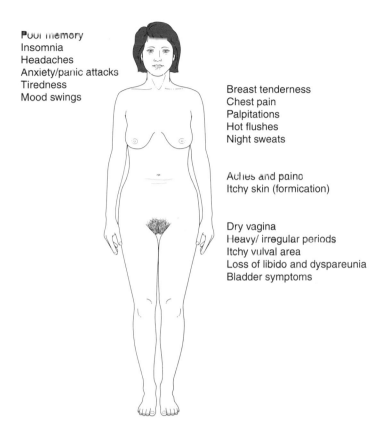

Poor memory
Insomnia
Headaches
Anxiety/panic attacks
Tiredness
Mood swings

Breast tenderness
Chest pain
Palpitations
Hot flushes
Night sweats

Aches and pains
Itchy skin (formication)

Dry vagina
Heavy/ irregular periods
Itchy vulval area
Loss of libido and dyspareunia
Bladder symptoms

Figure 2.1 Summary of typical symptoms associated with the menopause.

However, it is estimated that up to 75% of postmenopausal women do experience acute symptoms, often starting before menstruation even stops and sometimes continuing for many years afterwards. Many symptoms are entirely self-limiting with no effect other than mild discomfort to a woman, whereas others become so distressing that they may upset a woman's life substantially (McKinlay & Jeffreys 1974, Samsioe et al 1985):

- ◆ 25% of women continue to experience symptoms for 5 years
- ◆ 5% of women are still experiencing symptoms many years after the menopause
- ◆ 51% of symptomatic women describe their symptoms as 'severe'.

The average length of time for which a woman experiences symptoms is around 2 years. Symptoms come and go in some women, whereas others have symptoms more persistently. The severity of symptoms also varies, both among women and even within an individual's own experience (Fig. 2.2). Two women may experience the same degree of symptoms, yet one will cope while another finds them disruptive to her life. This will depend on her job and her lifestyle as well as her attitude to the symptoms and how well she can cope with them.

VASOMOTOR SYMPTOMS

The **hot flush** is probably the symptom that is most widely recognized as being related to the menopause. Almost all women and many men would be able to associate the hot flush with 'the change'. Hot flushes are extremely common, although their frequency and intensity will vary greatly between individuals.

Women describe a hot flush as a feeling of intense heat, sometimes accompanied by sweating, starting in the chest area and rising through the neck and face. When flushes occur at night, they often manifest as **night sweats**, causing a woman to awaken feeling most uncomfortable and very hot and sweaty. These can continue for many months, night after night, leaving the woman feeling both physically tired and emotionally drained as a result of lack of sleep

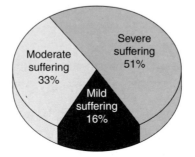

Figure 2.2 Severity of symptoms in menopausal women in the UK.

(Fig. 2.3). This can cause stress in a relationship between partners, particularly if it continues for a long time.

The actual cause of hot flushes is unclear. They do not seem to be related to specific levels of oestrogen in the blood, but rather to the rate of change (Teede & Burger 1998). This would explain why they are most common in the early stages of the climacteric – the time of greatest hormonal upheaval.

Flushes and sweats are not life threatening but they can be very distressing. Many women are affected at work, causing embarrassment and difficulty. Home and leisure activities are also affected. Fortunately, flushes respond well to hormone replacement therapy (HRT) (Coope et al 1975). Within 2–3 weeks of starting treatment, flushes and sweats should be improved, and if an adequate dose of oestrogen is given they should disappear altogether. Other methods of relieving flushes and sweats are discussed in Chapter 8. Hot flushes can be worsened by:

◆ hot and spicy foods
◆ alcohol intake

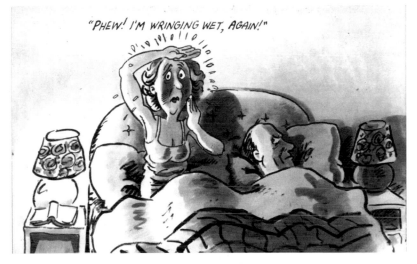

Figure 2.3 Night sweats can lead to a woman feeling physically and emotionally drained. From slide set 'Understanding the Menopause', with permission of Wyeth Laboratories.

◆ cigarette smoking
◆ caffeine intake
◆ hot weather.

Hot flushes may be associated with **palpitations**, which can lead to symptoms of anxiety as women worry that there is something seriously wrong with their heart.

MUSCLE AND JOINT PAINS

Many women complain of generalized aches and pains around the time of the climacteric. It is often impossible to say whether such symptoms are in fact hormonally related or whether this is an age-related phenomenon. There is no evidence that HRT directly relieves joint pains, although improvements in well-being may lead to a general improvement in quality of life (Coope 1996).

SKIN SYMPTOMS

Women on HRT often describe a change in their skin elasticity which may be due to a beneficial effect on the collagen content. Changes in the skin at the time of the menopause can lead to:

◆ loss of elasticity and suppleness
◆ dry skin
◆ formication (intense tingling or sensation of crawling on the skin).

BLADDER SYMPTOMS

Symptoms such as pruritus, pain and dysuria are frequent in post-menopausal women. However, it is difficult to differentiate between symptoms that are genuinely hormone related and those that are caused by general ageing factors. It is true that women are often more aware of their symptoms at around the time of the meno-pause, with one study showing that 50% of women attending a menopause clinic had urinary symptoms (Versi 1995). However, whether the menopause itself has actually caused the problems is unclear. Oestrogen and progesterone receptors have been found in the urethra and the bladder, so it is likely that they will be sensitive to hormone changes (Versi & Cardozo 1988). Typical bladder symptoms are:

◆ stress incontinence
◆ frequency of micturition
◆ urgency of micturition
◆ nocturia.

Women are often embarrassed to talk about bladder problems, so sympathetic questioning may be required. A trial of oestrogen therapy may be beneficial.

Nocturia, urgency and urge incontinence may be helped by oestrogen, whereas the condition of genuine stress incontinence is not thought to be helped by oestrogen (Versi 1994). Referral for urodynamic studies should be considered for women whose bladder symptoms are severe enough to affect their normal daily activities. Women should not feel that such symptoms must simply be tolerated as an inevitable part of middle age.

SEXUAL FUNCTION

Women attending menopause clinics often complain of sexual problems (Graziottin 1998). However, few studies have assessed sexual function in a general population at the menopause transition. Sarrel (1988) has described changes that are commonly experienced:

◆ decreased sexual desire
◆ diminished sexual response
◆ loss of libido
◆ orgasmic difficulty.

Dennerstein et al (2000) describe a longitudinal study of 354 Australian women and their experiences. They found:

◆ decline in sexual interest
◆ dyspareunia
◆ decreased occurrence of intercourse.

This study described how factors other than hormonal ones are also powerful in their effect on sexual function during the menopausal transition:

◆ women's expectations of sexual behaviour
◆ general well-being
◆ stress
◆ presence of bothersome symptoms
◆ feelings for partner.

Both hormonal and non-hormonal factors will influence sexual function at the time of the menopause.

Oestrogen lack

Declining oestrogen levels at the time of the menopause and thereafter (unless HRT is taken) result in profound changes to the vagina and vulval areas. Atrophic changes result in a shorter, less elastic vagina with less vascularity and a thinner and more easily irritated epithelium – **atrophic vaginitis**. This can lead to **vaginal dryness** and **dyspareunia** (painful intercourse). This inevitably stops a woman from enjoying lovemaking to the full and can result in both physical and psychological problems. Vaginal secretions diminish and the vagina becomes more susceptible to infection because of a changing pH. Changes in the vagina due to oestrogen deficiency are:

◆ increased pH – less resistance to infection
◆ decreased blood flow
◆ loss of elasticity
◆ shortens in length
◆ loss of muscle tone
◆ decreased cervical secretion.

Replacing oestrogen either systemically or locally will help to maintain vaginal lubrication and assist in making sexual intercourse more comfortable.

Anxiety

If sexual intercourse is painful or results in bleeding, a woman may become anxious and tense, which will make her next attempt at intercourse less successful. A cycle can be established, such as that shown in Figure 2.4.

Body image

The climacteric can be a time when a woman has to confront the fact that she is ageing. The cessation of menstruation is tangible evidence that the reproductive phase is over. For some women this is a relief: contraception is no longer required and sex can be enjoyed simply for its own sake. Women with this attitude may expect to continue a satisfying sex life well into their post-menopausal years and, indeed, continuing sexual intercourse after the menopause may in itself help to prevent atrophic changes (Leiblum et al 1983).

Other women consider the menopause to be a step towards old age, a time of deterioration in health, both physical and sexual. Such an attitude can produce a psychological barrier to continuing

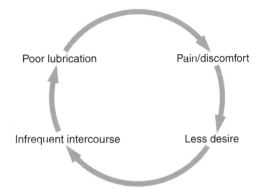

Figure 2.4 Cycle demonstrating sexual difficulties.

sexual relations. Negative self-image can contribute to a sense of feeling non-sexual and therefore to a loss of desire for sexual activity (Graziottin 1998). This is discussed further in Chapter 5.

The couple relationship

Problems with sexual activity around mid life are not necessarily a simple result of hormonal changes in the individual woman. A male partner may also be developing problems such as erectile difficulty or loss of desire. Physical attraction and intimacy may be affected by bodily changes attributed to the ageing process as well as to hormones. These may be contributing to a less than satisfying sexual relationship. Satisfaction within the relationship, emotional stability and psychological well-being will all contribute to a healthy and satisfying sex life. If a problem exists it will probably exist for both partners, although they may be affected in different ways. On the other hand, a new partner may contribute to an increase in libido and satisfaction in the context of a new relationship.

Psychosexual counselling

Some couples will need specific counselling and help in their relationship. Such counselling will involve (Sarrel 1988):

◆ careful and attentive listening
◆ provision of information about sexual function
◆ reassurance
◆ suggestions for improving communication about feelings
◆ encouragement to re-establish sexual activity when appropriate.

For most women, a combination of counselling, reassurance and HRT, if appropriate, will be sufficient for a couple to resolve sexual difficulties. A few women may need referral to a sex therapist for more in-depth treatment.

PSYCHOLOGICAL SYMPTOMS

In addition to physical symptoms, some women experience emotional or psychological symptoms around the time of the menopause. Many women do not understand that such feelings may occur and become very anxious about them. Typical psychological symptoms are:

◆ panic attacks
◆ poor memory
◆ lack of concentration
◆ irritability
◆ mood swings
◆ anxiety
◆ depressed mood
◆ fatigue.

Despite many studies, it has proved difficult to ascertain whether these symptoms are truly endocrine effects or whether they arise as a result of compounding factors affecting a woman at this time. Mid life is often a time of social and emotional upheaval and the following may be contributory factors to psychological symptoms:

◆ marriage difficulties
◆ divorce
◆ children leaving home
◆ change in work or home responsibilities
◆ death or illness in the family.

These factors are discussed more fully in Chapter 5.

Nevertheless, some studies have shown that minor psychological complaints can correlate to fluctuating oestrogen levels (Ballinger 1975, Montgomery et al 1987). Hunter et al (1986) showed that, in a study of 850 women, depressed mood and sleep problems were more common in the perimenopausal era than premenopausally. This confirmed the work of earlier studies (Ballinger 1975, Thompson et al 1973).

The 'domino effect' has also been described (Landau & Milan 1996). Psychological effects may arise from the physical symptoms of the climacteric.

It is unlikely that all psychological symptoms attributed to 'the change' are truly hormone related, but rather that there is an interaction between physical and psychological factors affecting women at this time (Table 2.1). Women may be more prone to psychological symptoms during the climacteric if they have a past history of psychiatric disease or if they experience difficulty in coping with stress (Hunter 1988).

Effect of HRT on psychological symptoms

HRT may help psychological symptoms as well as physical ones. Campbell & Whitehead (1977) found that oestrogen was significantly more effective than placebo in alleviating symptoms such as anxiety, poor memory, irritability and insomnia. Some of the women in this study did not experience hot flushes so the assumption is that the beneficial effect was direct rather than through the domino effect. Women with severe physical symptoms, relieved by HRT, often describe psychological improvement as well, highlighting the obvious interaction between the physical and the psychological.

Psychological symptoms may cause a woman great anxiety, so reassurance and explanations are an important part of her care. Non-hormonal therapies for the relief of psychological symptoms are discussed in Chapter 8.

Table 2.1 Summary of typical effects of oestrogen deficiency	
	Effects
Short term	Flushes/sweats
	Psychological complaints
	Insomnia
	Joint pains
Intermediate	Vaginal symptoms
	Bladder symptoms
	Sexual difficulties
Long term	Osteoporosis
	Cardiovascular disease

The effects of menopausal symptoms are often underestimated by health professionals. Women often say that they do not feel they are taken seriously by their doctor or that they (the patient) do not want to 'trouble' the doctor over something that is distressing but not life threatening. However, for some women these symptoms will affect not just their home life, but their work and their relationships too. It is therefore important that women are encouraged at least to discuss their symptoms, even if they ultimately decide to persevere with them and not take HRT. Reassurance that typical symptoms are normal is sometimes enough. Lack of information and knowledge will lead only to further anxiety. Women need more information both about typical menopausal symptoms and about treatment that may be available for them.

Menopause and depression

There is considerable debate as to whether mood changes and psychological symptoms are linked to menopause or whether the psychosocial factors discussed above play a more important role. There is also controversy regarding the incidence of depression at menopause and whether declining oestrogen levels are in fact associated with an increased risk of negative mood change in women (Collins 1998). The menopause generally occurs around mid life for women, which is often perceived as a time of increased stress. The interaction between physiological and psychological factors is probably important in determining a woman's reaction to hormonal change. Social and family factors have been shown to be more important in the aetiology of psychological symptoms than changing hormone levels (McKinlay et al 1987), although other studies have shown that women who experience a surgical menopause have more psychological symptomatology than those undergoing a natural menopause (Kaufert et al 1992, Khastigar & Studd 1998). It is not clear whether the menopause itself predisposes to depression, but it is difficult to isolate the causal factor when there may be so many other influences on a woman at this time (Nicol-Smith 1996).

REFERENCES

Ballinger CB (1975) Psychiatric morbidity and the menopause screening of general population: sample. *Br. Med J.* **3**: 344.

Campbell S, Whitehead MI (1977) Oestrogen therapy and the menopausal syndrome. *Clin. Obstet. Gynaecol.* **4**: 31–47.

Collins A (1998) Depression and the menopausal transition. In: Studd JW (ed.) *The Management of the Menopause, Annual Review*, pp. 13–18. Parthenon, London.

Coope J (1996) Hormonal and nonhormonal interventions for menopausal symptoms. *Maturitas* **23**: 159–168.

Coope J, Thompson JM, Poller L (1975) Effect of 'natural oestrogen' replacement therapy on menopausal symptoms and blood clotting. *Br. Med. J.* **4**: 139.

Dennerstein L, Lehert P, Burger H, Garamszerg C, Dudley E (2000) Menopause and sexual functioning. In: Studd JW (ed.) *The Management of the Menopause, Millennium Review*, pp. 203–210. Parthenon, London.

Graziottin A (1998) Sexuality and the menopause In: Studd JW (ed.) *The Management of the Menopause, Annual Review*, pp. 49–58. Parthenon, London.

Hunter M (1988) Psychological aspects of the climacteric. In: Studd JWW, Whitehead MI (eds) *The Menopause*, pp. 55–64. Blackwell Scientific, Oxford.

Hunter MS, O'Dea I (1997) Menopause: bodily changes and multiple meanings. In: Ussher JM (ed.) *Body Talk: The Material and Discursive Regulation of Sexuality, Madness and Reproduction.* Routledge, London.

Hunter M, Battersby R, Whitehead MI (1986) Relationships between psychological symptoms, somatic complaints and menopause status. *Maturitas* **8**: 217–218.

Kaufert PA, Gilbert P, Tate R (1992) The Manitoba Project: a re-examination of the link between menopause and depression. *Maturitas* **14**: 143–155.

Khastigar G, Studd J (1998) Hysterectomy, ovarian failure and depression. *Menopause* **5**: 113–122.

Landau C, Milan FB (1996) Assessment and treatment of depression during the menopause: a preliminary report. *Menopause* **3**: 201–207.

Leiblum SR, Bachmann GA, Kemmann E et al (1983) Vaginal atrophy in the postmenopausal woman. *J. Am. Med. Assoc.* **249**: 2195–2198.

McKinlay J, McKinlay S, Brambilla D (1987) The relative contribution of endocrine and social circumstances to depression in middle aged women. *J. Health Soc. Behav.* **28**: 345–363.

McKinlay SM, Jeffreys M (1974) The menopausal syndrome. *Br. J. Prevent. Med.* **28**: 108.

Montgomery JC, Appleby L, Brincat M et al (1987) Effects of oestrogen and testosterone implant therapy on psychological disorders in the climacteric. *Lancet* **i**: 297.

Nicol-Smith L (1996) Causality, menopause and depression: a critical review of the literature. *Br. Med. J.* **313**: 1129–1132.

Samsioe G, Bryman I, Ivansson E (1985) Some anthropological aspects of the climacteric syndrome. *Acta Obstet. Gynaecol. Scand. Suppl.* **130**: 5.

Sarrel PM (1988) Sexuality. In: Studd JWW, Whitehead MI (eds) *The Menopause*, pp. 65–75. Blackwell Scientific, Oxford.

Teede H, Burger HG (1998) The menopausal transition. In: Studd JW (ed.) *The Management of the Menopause, Annual Review*, pp. 1–12. Parthenon, London.

Thompson B, Hart SA, Durno D (1973) Menopausal age and symptomatology in general practice. *J. Biol. Soc. Sci.* **5**: 71–82.

Versi E (1994) Ageing and hormonal changes of the bladder and urethra. *Curr. Prob. Obstet. Gynaecol. Fertil.* **17**: 193–232.

Versi E (1995) Urinary disorders and the menopause. *Menopause* **2**: 89–95.

Versi E, Cardozo LD (1988) Oestrogens and the lower urinary tract function. In: Studd JWW, Whitehead MI (eds) *The Menopause*, pp. 76–84. Blackwell Scientific, Oxford.

3

Long-term Consequences of Oestrogen Deficiency

It is probably true to say that women are most concerned about the immediate effects of the menopause on their lives – the symptoms, whether physical or psychological. When symptoms become disruptive to their lives, they seek help. Hormone replacement therapy (HRT) looks more attractive to a woman when she can see the tangible benefits she may enjoy. Yet, from a medical perspective, these symptoms are usually harmless, however inconvenient they may be at the time. They can cause a lot of discomfort, embarrassment and heartache, but are seldom life threatening in themselves. Many will disappear spontaneously if left untreated, although it may take several years. For many women, months or even years of their lives will be spoiled, so it is important that even short-term HRT is made available to them if appropriate.

In the long term, however, women's bodies do change as a result of the menopause. The skeleton and the cardiovascular system are the most readily identified as changing after the menopause, but it is possible that many other body systems are affected. One area that is being researched at present is the brain, in relation to **Alzheimer's disease**.

ALZHEIMER'S DISEASE

For many, one of the most feared consequences of ageing is dementia, most commonly caused by Alzheimer's disease. This is a progressive neurodegenerative disorder; its prevalence among the elderly doubles about every 4–5 years (Jorm et al 1987). Even after adjusting for age, women appear to be at greater risk than men (Henderson 1998).

Support for a protective role of oestrogen replacement comes from epidemiological studies. An example is the Leisure World Study in California (Paginini-Hill & Henderson 1996): women who had used oestrogen therapy were shown to have a one-third reduction in their risk of Alzheimer's disease compared with women who had never used oestrogen. Henderson and colleagues (1996) observed that women actually suffering from Alzheimer's disease and receiving oestrogen had better cognitive ability than those not using oestrogen. Others have investigated this, but most studies are small, uncontrolled and of short duration. The results of studies such as these are promising and point to the need for further prospective studies of HRT in postmenopausal women with and without Alzheimer's disease.

OSTEOPOROSIS

Osteoporosis is not a new problem. However, as life expectancy improves and with more and more elderly people living in our society, awareness of this disease is becoming important. The National Service Framework for Older People, provided by the Department of Health (2001), includes a major section on osteoporosis, with detailed standards on how osteoporosis should be diagnosed, treated and prevented in people aged over 50 years. Although the prevalence of osteoporosis among men is increasing too, it is principally women who need a greater understanding of the disease and how they might be affected. Oestrogen deficiency is the main cause of osteoporosis in women, arising as a consequence of the menopause, although it is often not until many years later that the effects are seen. It is the more elderly women who commonly experience fractures relating to osteoporosis (Grimley-Evans et al 1979). Yet, if the disease is to be prevented, measures need to be taken at a much earlier stage in life. While it is never too late to try to minimize the effects of osteoporosis, it is wise to start early and in particular to consider the time of the menopause as an important stage in the development of the disease. This section will look at what osteoporosis is, how it may be prevented, and what interventions may help.

Definition

'Osteoporosis is a systemic skeletal disease characterised by low bone mass and microarchitectural deterioration of bone tissue, with a consequent increase in bone fragility and susceptibility to fractures' (World Health Organization 1994)

Osteoporosis is a condition in which the structure of the bone (or 'bone mass') weakens to such an extent that the risk of fracture is greatly increased. These fractures occur not as a result of major trauma, but often following trivial accidents or even during everyday activities. For example, an elderly woman might simply step off the kerb and fracture a hip, or bend down in the garden and suffer a spinal fracture. Women at risk of such fractures are said to have osteoporosis even if they have not yet experienced a fracture. The categories of osteoporosis are defined in terms of measured bone mineral density and fracture (Table 3.1).

Table 3.1 Definition of osteoporosis according to World Health Organization criteria (WHO 1994)

Diagnosis	Bone mineral density (T score, standard deviation units)
Normal	< 1 SD
Osteopenia	Between 1 and 2.5 SD
Osteoporosis	> 2.5 SD
Severe osteoporosis	> 2.5 SD and presence of one or more fragility fractures

It is interesting to note that the values shown in Table 3.1 are defined principally for caucasians. It may be that normal values for other ethnic groups are different, requiring different interpretation and interventions, but until further research is available this reference should be used (Kanis & Gluer 2000). There is concern that measurements made at one site may not correlate to measurements made at another site, although advances have been made to standardize hip and spine measurements between different equipment (Kanis & Gluer 2000). The available evidence suggests that the diagnostic use of T scores should be reserved for dual-energy absorptiometry of the hip (Kanis & Gluer 2000).

The ageing process

In the mature adult, skeletal size is neither increasing nor decreasing. During childhood and young adulthood there is a net increase in bone density, resulting in skeletal growth. At around the age of 35 years, peak bone mass is achieved and less bone formation takes place. This results in an overall decline in bone density as we get older (Fig. 3.1). This process occurs in both men and women, and is related to age (Riggs et al 1982). Women also demonstrate an additional rapid decline in bone density around the time of the menopause and for several years afterwards (Melton et al 1992, Stevenson et al 1989). It is this sudden decrease in bone density that can cause a woman to fall below the so-called **fracture threshold** later in life.

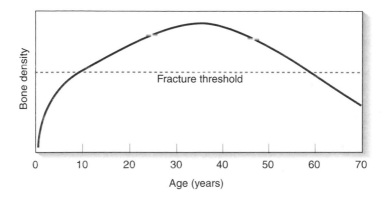

Figure 3.1 Changes of bone density with age.

One aim of any osteoporosis prevention strategy is to prevent bone density from falling below this fracture threshold, thus ideally preventing the occurrence of fractures. Long-term strategies also include trying to improve peak bone mass in young adults. This means that the prevention of osteoporosis should be taken seriously throughout life.

Normal bone structure

Bone is a living part of the body, being continually removed and renewed. In adults this activity is accounted for largely by **bone remodelling**. Bone remodelling comprises the process of bone resorption followed by bone formation and provides a mechanism for self-repair and adaptation to stress. There is a linked cycle of bone resorption followed by bone renewal. **Osteoclasts** lie on bone surfaces or in pits and create cavities in the bone, which may take up to 2 months to remineralize. They are the cells responsible for the synthesis of collagen and other bone proteins. **Osteoblasts** are the bone-forming cells which replace and renew bone. These coupled functional units of osteoclasts and osteoblasts have been called bone multicellular units (BMUs). They are asynchronous, so resorption at one site is balanced by formation at another, with no net weakening of the skeleton.

If bone resorption exceeds bone formation, low bone mass occurs. Rate of turnover in bone will also influence how rapidly this occurs. The loss of bone mass that results in osteoporosis is the result of the daily rate of bone resorption exceeding the rate of bone formation (Woolfe & St John Dixon 1998). This has typically been demonstrated in women who have undergone oophorectomy (Stepan et al 1987). In osteoporosis, not only is the number of osteoclasts increased, but the depth of resorption may be greater. The number of osteoblasts is increased, but performance may be less than normal, after the menopause (Kanis 1994).

Bone is not a solid structure, but is made up of a network of fibres, criss-crossing each other to maintain strength. Osteoporotic bone has less strength because the criss-cross structures become broken or decayed, causing the overall structure to be weakened (Fig. 3.2).

The strength of the skeleton at a given time will depend on the **bone density**, or **bone mass**. This will be at its peak at around the mid-thirties, declining gradually thereafter. Peak bone mass (i.e. the maximum to be achieved) is influenced by the following factors:

◆ race
◆ genetic factors
◆ hormonal influences

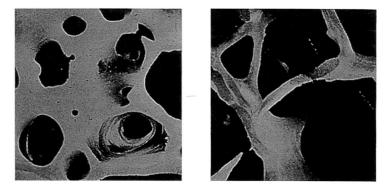

Figure 3.2 Electron micrograph showing normal and osteoporotic bone. Reproduced from Dempster et al (1986) with permission. © Elsevier Science Inc.

◆ nutrition
◆ smoking
◆ use of certain medications.

Incidence

Osteoporotic fractures are extremely common. Each year there are approximately 200 000 fractures of the hip, wrist and spine, the majority of which are likely to have been caused by osteoporosis. The three commonest sites for fracture as a result of osteoporosis are the wrist, spine and hip (Fig. 3.3).

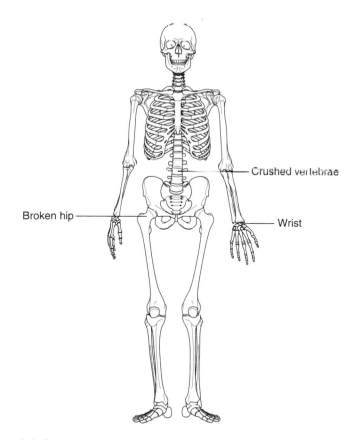

Figure 3.3 Common sites for osteoporotic fracture.

Wrist

Each year there are about 40 000 cases of fracture of the distal fore-arm, often resulting from a fall on to an outstretched hand. They may occur premenopausally in women who have a low bone density, and may be considered an 'early warning sign' of osteoporosis. The rate of these fractures rises in women after the age of 50 years until around the age of 65 years. There is no corresponding increase seen in men at this age. After the age of 65 years there appears to be no further rise in the rate of these fractures among women (Stevenson & Marsh 1992).

Hip

The incidence of hip fracture among elderly women is remarkably high; these fractures are potentially very serious. Treatment of hip fractures is by surgical fixation, which carries the immediate risk associated with general anaesthesia and the longer-term risks associated with immobility in an already elderly or frail person. Surgical complications arise in about one-third of patients and long-term morbidity is high. Only a minority of women regain their former mobility (Melton 1993). The incidence of hip fractures is likely to increase as a result of a rise in the number of elderly people in the population (Grimley-Evans 1990).

Spine

Vertebral fractures occur when osteoporosis causes the vertebral bodies to collapse, causing a 'wedging' or crush fracture. The incidence of these fractures is difficult to assess because they often occur silently and are demonstrated only on X-ray at a much later stage. Vertebral fractures often occur spontaneously or after only minimal trauma, such as lifting or sneezing (Kanis 1994). It has been estimated that only one-third of such fractures are brought to medical attention at the actual time of fracture (Grimley-Evans 1990). Sudden acute fractures of the vertebra cause intense pain, requiring urgent medical help. The so-called 'dowager's hump', or **kyphosis**, arises after repeated vertebral fractures causing loss of height and pain. The occurrence of a vertebral fracture is an

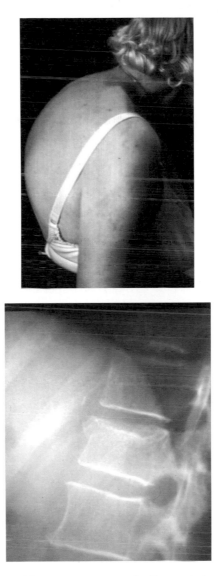

Figure 3.4 Woman with severe osteoporosis. By permission of Mcdipic/Peter Stott.

independent risk fracture for further fractures. Over 10 years more than 80% of patients will have a recurrent fracture and three-quarters will go on to lose 10 cm in height (Kanis 1994) (Fig. 3.4).

Causes

Osteoporosis can be caused by various factors. Peak bone mass is achieved by early adulthood and is largely genetically predetermined. Lifestyle factors such as diet and exercise may also influence the development of the skeleton (Kandlers et al 1984, Kanis & Passmore 1989). Race is also an influencing factor: black women have a greater bone density than whites and Asians (Woolfe & St John Dixon 1998).

Whether or not a woman suffers osteoporosis will depend not only on how good a peak bone mass she achieves as a young adult but also on the rate at which she loses bone density later in life. Around the time of the menopause, the rate of bone loss averages 2% per year over the next 5–10 years, and then declines. An early menopause is associated with a low bone mass and accelerated risk of fracture (Richelson et al 1984). Loss of bone after the menopause is not uniform. On this basis, postmenopausal women have been categorized into so-called 'normal' and 'fast' bone losers (Hansen et al 1991). A woman might achieve an excellent peak bone mass, but subsequently lose bone very quickly, putting her at as much risk as a woman who achieves a low peak bone mass but who then loses mass at a much slower rate. Factors that determine the rates of bone loss are not completely understood, but are discussed below (see Risk factors).

Whilst osteoporosis is commonly a result of oestrogen deficiency at the time of the menopause, it may also occur as a result of the following factors:

◆ corticosteroid therapy (above 7.5 mg prednisolone daily or equivalent dose, on a regular basis)
◆ hyperparathyroidism
◆ Cushing's syndrome
◆ some malignant diseases
◆ long-term immobilization
◆ excessive exercise, as in athletes or ballet dancers
◆ chronic hepatic or renal failure
◆ rheumatoid arthritis.

Risk factors

Various risk factors have been identified that are thought to predict those women who may be at an increased risk of developing osteoporosis and therefore who may experience fractures later in life. Identifying the women at risk would mean that intervention strategies could be targeted, and those most likely to be at risk of fracture in the future could receive treatment. Common risk factors are:

◆ low bodyweight
◆ previous low trauma fracture
◆ family history of hip fracture
◆ early menopause
◆ prolonged amenorrhoea
◆ long-term corticosteroid therapy.

Studies have shown, however, that risk factors such as these are not good predictors of future risk of fracture. In the absence of other more accurate methods of predicting risk, these factors may sometimes be the only indication of whether a woman is potentially at risk. The risk of fracture is inversely related to bone mineral density (Cummings et al 1993), so it is considered far more accurate to measure the bone density in order to predict future risk of fracture.

Measuring bone density

Dual-energy X-ray absorptiometry

Measurements of bone mineral density at the spine and hip using **dual-energy X-ray absorptiometry (DXA)** (see Fig. 3.5) are currently considered the 'gold standard' for diagnosis of osteoporosis (Kanis & Gluer 2000). Such measurements are both accurate and precise, and involve exposure to very low doses of ionizing radiation. Traditionally DXA measurements have been made at the lumbar spine and the proximal femur, and these are thought to be the most useful in diagnosis. Measurements can also be made at peripheral sites such as the distal forearm, although the predictive capacity appears to be slightly less than that of measurements at the hip and spine (National Osteoporosis Society 1998). A single

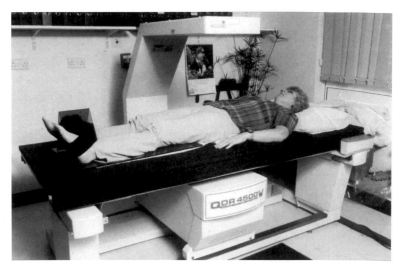

Figure 3.5 DEXA machine, courtesy of the Medical Illustration Department, Northwick Park Hospital, Harrow.

measurement at any site is useful as a one-time assessment of fracture risk at that site (Hodgson & Conrad Johnston 1996). Bone mineral density at any site should be used in conjunction with a clinical assessment of other risk factors and a medical history.

Quantitative computed tomography (QCT)

QCT is used to measure bone density in the spine. It uses larger doses of radiation and is considerably more expensive than other methods. It is often used for research purposes.

Ultrasonography

Ultrasonography can be used to measure bone density in the heel. Currently there are no established criteria for the definition of osteoporosis using heel ultrasonography, so the use of it cannot be compared with X-ray absorptiometry. A low bone density in the heel appears to correlate with a low density in the hip or spine, but further research is required (Stewart et al 1996). Potentially this simple method of measurement could be used widely as a tool for assessing the risk of osteoporosis or for identifying women who require further investigation, which will usually include DXA (National Osteoporosis Society 1998)

Why measure bone density?

Measurement of bone density at around the time of the menopause will help to identify whether a woman is at risk of fracture in later life (Cummings et al 1993). A further scan 18–24 months later will also help to assess the actual rate of bone loss over this period of time. Such measurements are particularly useful for women who are reluctant to take HRT but are concerned about osteoporosis. If a bone density measurement clearly shows an increased risk, it is much easier for the woman to understand the need for HRT and will help her to make an informed decision. Repeat scans can also encourage a woman to remain on therapy because there is tangible evidence of the benefits. In high-risk women measurement of bone density can ensure that the doses of treatment given are sufficient for protection in that individual woman.

So far, there is insufficient evidence to support widespread screening of all women, as a cost-effective and efficient exercise. Meanwhile on an individual basis, bone density measurements can be helpful, particularly in highlighting those women who would not consider medical intervention except for prevention of osteoporosis.

On the NHS?

The Department of Health (DoH) supports the use of bone density as a means of assessing patients on an individual basis and has recommended that facilities should be available (DoH 1994). Osteoporosis is included in the National Service Framework for Older People (DoH 2001), which sets standards and a framework for best practice relating to osteoporosis in older people.

To clarify who would benefit from bone density measurement, some health authorities have drawn up clear guidelines as to who to refer. Categories of women who may be referred for bone densitometry include (Lee 2000):

- Women at the menopause in whom the decision to take HRT would be affected by the results of bone mineral densitometry
- Those who have osteopenia (low bone mass) diagnosed on spinal radiography
- People on long-term corticosteroid therapy (7.5 mg or more of prednisolone)
- Women with a history of one osteoporosis-related fracture
- Women with diseases known to cause bone loss
- Women with low body mass index ($< 19\,\text{kg/m}^2$)
- Women with early menopause (natural or surgical) or prolonged amenorrhoea
- Women with a strong family history of osteoporosis (e.g. mother with hip fracture)
- To monitor response to therapy.

The role of calcium

Many women believe that if they simply take extra calcium at the time of the menopause they will prevent osteoporosis. Calcium, like all vitamins and minerals, is an essential part of a healthy diet. The majority of women who eat a well-balanced diet will not benefit simply by taking calcium supplements. Calcium supplementation is usually considered to be an adjunct to other management strategies, including lifestyle and exercise changes. Women with low calcium intake or malabsorption may require calcium and vitamin D supplements. Studies have shown that elderly women who have a poor calcium intake may benefit from calcium supplements and see a slight rise in bone mineral density (Dawson-Hughes et al 1991).

A healthy diet should be encouraged and women who eat very few dairy products may be deficient in calcium if they are not taking it in other foods. These women should be advised about the possible need for dietary supplements (see Chapter 8). Recommended daily allowances for calcium are shown in Table 3.2.

Table 3.2 Recommended calcium intake, based on the Department of Health Committee on Medical Aspects of Food and Nutrition Policy (COMA) 1998 recommendations

	Calcium (mg/day)
Adults	
Men	700
Women	700
Teenagers (11–18 years)	
Boys	1000
Girls	800
Children	
1–3 years	350
4–6 years	450
7–10 years	550
Pregnant and breastfeeding women	700

Exercise

Regular weight-bearing exercise, such as walking or jogging, produces a small increase in bone density in postmenopausal women (Chow et al 1987, Gleeson et al 1990). However it cannot prevent the rapid bone loss experienced at the time of the menopause. Exercise improves flexibility, muscle tone and general fitness, perhaps reducing the likelihood of a fall.

Exercise is always to be recommended as a positive lifestyle change. It needs to be consistent and regular if benefits are to be noticed. Weight-bearing exercise, such as dancing, tennis, badminton and walking, for 30 minutes at least four times a week is recommended for promoting healthy bone. Women may need to build up to this gradually and, as with all exercise programmes, they should seek the advice of their GP before starting a new programme. Whilst activities specific to each site will help bone strength, aerobic exercise will encourage suppleness, strength, balance and coordination.

Excessive exercise such as that undertaken by athletes or ballet dancers in training is harmful to bone, resulting in a low premenopausal bone density, which will increase the risk of fracture in later life, particularly following a further rapid loss at the time of the menopause (Drinkwater et al 1984). This is likely to be due to low oestrogen levels which often occur in these women, leading to prolonged episodes of amenorrhoea or oligomenorrhoea.

HRT AND OSTEOPOROSIS

HRT remains the first treatment of choice for women without contraindications who want to treat or prevent osteoporosis. Retrospective studies have shown that 5 years' use of oestrogen therapy is associated with a halving of the risk of hip fracture (Hillard et al 1994, Lindsay et al 1980). Vertebral fracture risk is also reduced (Ettinger et al 1985, Naessen et al 1990). These results indicate that, when considering the use of HRT as a protection against osteoporosis, long-term treatment is recommended. Women should be aware that taking HRT for only a few months is unlikely to confer much benefit. Oestrogens may reduce the rate of fracture by increasing mobility and dexterity as well as the known direct effects of oestrogen on bone cells.

The precise mechanism by which oestrogens act on osteoblasts and osteoclasts to protect the skeleton is unclear. In osteoporosis, bone resorption outpaces bone formation, a process that is decreased by about 50% during oestrogen therapy (Steiniche et al 1989). The arrest on bone loss will last as long as treatment continues (Kanis 1994).

Studies have demonstrated that implants, patches and tablets all have the effect of preserving bone density, although the required dose of each varies (Stevenson et al 1990). It is important to note that the dose of oestrogen required for prevention of bone loss may differ from that required for control of menopausal symptoms. A small number of women may need higher doses of oestrogen to prevent bone loss, but without bone density measurement it is difficult to know who they are.

When to start and stop HRT

For the greatest benefit to the skeleton, HRT should be started soon after the menopause and continue indefinitely, but this is not without risk (Ettinger et al 1985). However, if HRT is started later in life, there is evidence that substantial increases in bone density may be seen (Marx et al 1992). The difference in fracture risk at age 85 years among women who use lifelong HRT compared with those who commence at age 65 years may be small, because of the substantial increases seen in bone density in older women (Ettinger & Grady 1994). This suggests that active intervention in the elderly may still be useful.

When HRT is stopped, bone density declines, but usually at the same rate as immediately after the menopause. The rapid loss experienced at this time is thus delayed by the length of time a woman took HRT (Christiansen et al 1981, Kanis 1994, Lindsay et al 1978). Once a woman stops HRT she loses the protective effect and bone density will decrease – rapidly initially, then more slowly. It is not currently clear how long a woman would need to stay on HRT in order to see sustained benefit into her seventies and beyond.

OTHER TREATMENTS FOR OSTEOPOROSIS

Not all women want to take HRT and, indeed, some women are unable to because of medical contraindications. For these women, lifestyle changes are certainly worthwhile, particularly when considering preventing the disease. Women who already have osteoporosis may be offered alternative treatments:

◆ selective (o)estrogen receptor modulators (SERMs)
◆ calcitonin
◆ fluoride
◆ anabolic steroids
◆ bisphosphonates
◆ vitamin D.

Selective (o)estrogen receptor modulators

SERMs are a new class of drug compound that bind to and activate oestrogen receptors but which have different effects to conventional oestrogen replacement (Sato et al 1994). By offering tissue-specific activity, they may have significant potential for the prevention and treatment of diseases such as cancer, osteoporosis and heart disease. The precise mechanism of SERMs remains unclear, but the clinical effects on some organs have been closely studied. Raloxifene 60 mg daily (for the prevention and treatment of osteoporosis) prevents bone loss in postmenopausal women without causing endometrial proliferation. This means there is no associated bleeding as with many types of HRT. Raloxifene is not linked to an increased risk of breast cancer, indeed the Multiple Outcomes of Raloxifene Evaluation (MORE) study showed a reduction in the risk of oestrogen receptor-positive tumours (Cummings et al 1999). Raloxifene is generally well tolerated, with 10% of women experiencing new hot flushes in the first 6 months of treatment and a 7% increase in leg cramps (Ettinger et al 1999). The incidence of venous thrombosis is similar to that seen with conventional oestrogen use (Davies et al 1999).

Calcitonin

Calcitonin has been shown to maintain bone density, and in some studies actually to increase it (Gruber et al 1984). It works similarly to oestrogen, by inhibiting osteoclast activity. Its main drawback (apart from cost) is that in the UK it is currently administered by intramuscular injection. In some countries calcitonin is delivered by nasal spray. This form of treatment may offer an alternative to the woman at a high risk of osteoporosis but who cannot take HRT.

Fluoride

Fluoride has been used in the management of osteoporosis for more than 30 years but its use remains controversial (Kanis 1994). Fluoride stimulates bone formation, particularly in the spine, although the response rate between patients varies considerably

(Baud et al 1988). The usual dose is 20–60 mg daily, given with calcium supplementation. It has a number of side-effects, such as gastric upset and limb pains, so careful monitoring is essential. The risk of hip fracture may be increased in patients receiving fluoride (Riggs et al 1987).

Bisphosphonates

These are a group of drugs that are thought to work on bone in a similar way to HRT, yet are non-hormonal. **Disodium etidronate** was the first bisphosphonate to become available for treatment of established spinal osteoporosis. It is used as a cyclical therapy because continuous use would adversely affect bone mineralization. Etidronate 400 mg is given daily orally for 14 days, followed by calcium citrate 500 mg a day for a further 76 days, making a 90-day cycle, which is then repeated for 3–5 years. Etidronate should not be given to patients with renal impairment as it may induce osteomalacia (Kanis 1994).

Alendronate, another bisphosphonate, is available in a daily or weekly dosage regimen. It is licensed for the treatment and prevention of steroid-induced osteoporosis in men and women, and for the prevention and treatment of osteoporosis in postmenopausal women. The recommended dose is 5–10 mg, depending on the indication. The once-weekly dose is 70 mg for the prevention of postmenopausal osteoporosis.

Another available bisphosphonate is **risedronate**, given in a daily dose of 5 mg. This is licensed for the prevention and treatment of postmenopausal osteoporosis and steroid-induced osteoporosis in postmenopausal women.

Side-effects are rare with bisphosphonates; nausea and diarrhoea have been reported occasionally. Bisphosphonates are poorly absorbed from the gastrointestinal tract, so they should be taken with water and on an empty stomach. The manufacturers of both etidronate and alendronate include specific instructions to patients as to how to take the medication.

Vitamin D and derivatives

Women who are housebound or institutionalized and who rarely get outside into natural daylight may suffer from vitamin D deficiency. This can be corrected by giving supplements at a dose of 400–800 IU daily. However, research is contradictory as to whether vitamin D is of value in either the prevention or the treatment of osteoporosis. Calcitriol is a vitamin D derivative licensed for the treatment of postmenopausal osteoporosis. The recommended dose is 0.25 µg twice daily.

Isoflavones

Studies of the effects of isoflavones on bone health have produced mixed results. Gennari et al (1997) used ipriflavone 600 mg daily (a synthetic isoflavone) in comparison with placebo and saw a maintenance of bone density in women with low bone mass. Alexandersen et al (2001), however, showed no benefit to bone density in a similar study. Other research has shown a beneficial effect on bone using natural isoflavones (red clover) or soy-enriched bread (Dalais et al 1998, Nachitgall 2001). There is a need for further studies of isoflavones in relation to bone health.

PAIN RELIEF

The early stages of osteoporosis are not painful, but once fracture has occurred the condition can be very painful indeed. Hip fractures are treated surgically, but spinal fractures cannot be operated on, and for a few weeks after the fracture immense pain may be present. In some women the pain persists and becomes difficult to manage. When considering the treatment options, it is important to make a serious assessment of pain and suggest ways of relieving it. As well as conventional analgesia, the following could be considered:

◆ physiotherapy
◆ transcutaneous electrical nerve stimulation (TENS)
◆ acupuncture

- relaxation
- complementary therapies
- advice on coping with daily activities.

NATIONAL OSTEOPOROSIS SOCIETY

The National Osteoporosis Society, set up in 1986, is a national charity working towards improving care for osteoporosis sufferers. As well as providing general information and advice, it has produced a variety of booklets on subjects relating to osteoporosis. These include:

- general information about osteoporosis
- how to cope
- calcium guide
- fashion advice for sufferers
- treatments
- exercise and physiotherapy
- pain relief
- HRT.

The National Osteoporosis Society is an excellent source of accurate information for both patients and professionals. There is a scientific membership for medical professionals, providing details of conferences and study days as well as an update on research into osteoporosis and guidelines and protocols of care for professional use. See the Appendix for the address.

CARDIOVASCULAR DISEASE

In the past, most health education programmes relating to heart disease have been aimed at men. The stereotype 'executive flyer' who smokes, drinks, eats too many corporate lunches and never exercises has been targeted, with the aim of reducing the overall number of deaths from heart disease. Yet, heart disease is the major cause of death in women over the age of 60 years in the UK (DoH

1994). Over the past decade it has become clear that many physiological mechanisms are influenced by female sex hormones, including the cardiovascular system. The link between cardiovascular disease and female sex hormones was first suggested in the 1930s, with a link to the apparent protective effects of oestrogen on the cardiovascular system being made later. Initially the link was identified in women undergoing premature menopause by oophorectomy, and then in women experiencing natural menopause (Smolders & Van der Mooren 2000).

Significance of the menopause

While it recognized that ageing alone is a risk factor for cardiovascular disease, hormonal status clearly plays an important role in the incidence of cardiovascular disease in women. In early studies in the USA, it was demonstrated that, among groups of women in the same age band, those who were postmenopausal had a higher rate of cardiovascular disease than women who still had functioning ovaries (Gordon et al 1978). This was even more marked among the younger postmenopausal women (Rosenberg et al 1981).

HRT and cardiovascular disease

The menopause and its associated oestrogen loss appears to be a risk factor for the development of coronary heart disease (CHD) in women. Postmenopausal oestrogen therapy has been shown in a number of studies to have beneficial effects on cardiovascular risk factors, based on studies of animal and clinical models and observational studies of expected cardiovascular events (Nair & Herrington 2001). Opinion varies on the strength of the evidence that HRT reduces the risk of CHD. Large-scale retrospective studies, mainly from the USA, have shown a combined reduction in CHD risk of 42% in users of HRT (Grodstein & Stampfer 1995, Stampfer & Colditz 1991). Critics would argue that HRT users are not 'typical' women – they may have a high level of contact with medical professionals, they may have improved general health and they may already have been 'preselected' as being fit for oestrogen use. All of these factors, it is argued, lead to HRT users being at a lower risk of heart disease than non-users.

Three of the largest studies, the Nurses Health Study (Stampfer et al 1985), the Leisure World Study (Henderson et al 1991) and the Lipid Research Clinic Follow-up Study (Bush et al 1987), all showed that cardiovascular risk factors were similar in both users of oestrogen and non-users. These studies indicated that HRT appears to be a significant protective factor against heart disease in postmenopausal women. Some argue, however, that definite conclusions cannot be made from such studies and, until the results of large-scale randomized trials are available, there is no certainty of the preventive role of oestrogen in CHD. Large-scale studies are underway: the Women's Health Initiative in the USA and the Women's International Study of long Duration Oestrogen after Menopause (WISDOM) study in Europe.

Progestogens

The women in the large-scale studies that showed a protective benefit of HRT on the cardiovascular system used oestrogen-only therapy. With progestogens now routinely added to treatment regimens in the UK, the big question is whether the use of progestogen negates the cardiovascular benefits. Progestogens may have a less favourable effect on blood lipids, but this will vary according to the type and dose of progestogen (Lobo 1991). Few studies are available demonstrating the use of oestrogen–progestogen regimens, but a study in Sweden in 1992 showed a 50% reduction in the risk of myocardial infarction in users of a combined therapy (Falkeborn et al 1992). This indicates that the potential overall benefits of oestrogen are not necessarily lost with the addition of progestogen. The Postmenopausal Estrogen/Progestin Intervention (PEPI) Trial (1995) showed no evidence that adding progestogen to an oestrogen regimen reduces possible cardiovascular benefits.

Lipids

The lipid profile is a well-known predictor of cardiovascular risk. Accumulation of lipids in the arterial wall is considered to lead to atherosclerosis, probably accompanied by an inflammatory process (Ross 1999). After the menopause, changes occur in relation to lipids and lipoproteins that are thought to influence the onset of cardiovascular disease (Smolders et al 2000). Oestrogen therapy generally reduces levels of total cholesterol and low-density lipoproteins (LDLs) while increasing levels of high-density lipoproteins (HDLs). Transdermal therapy does not alter total HDL concentration, although there is a change in the subfractions of HDL. Higher concentrations of HDL are a protective factor in cardiovascular disease. Differences are seen with different progestogens (Smolders et al 2000).

The role of oestrogen therapy is important with regard to lipid changes, but it is thought unlikely that these changes fully explain the potential benefits of HRT on the cardiovascular system (Smolders et al 2000). Other ways in which HRT may be of benefit include:

◆ direct effects on blood vessel walls
◆ positive changes in insulin metabolism
◆ redistribution of body fat.

HRT and existing heart disease

Whether or not oestrogen therapy has a beneficial effect on women with existing heart disease is controversial. The Heart and Estrogen/Progestin Replacement Study (HERS) (Hulley et al 1998), using a combined oestrogen–progestogen regimen, showed no effect on CHD event rates and a trend towards an increase in CHD events in the first year of treatment. By years 4 and 5 this trend was reversed. Taking into account the known venous effects of oestrogen therapy, this suggests that more prolonged treatment may be required for cardiovascular benefit (Webb et al 2000). The Estrogen Replacement and Atherosclerosis (ERA) Study (Nair & Herrington 2001) supported the results of the HERS study, showing no benefit to postmenopausal women with CHD when conjugated oestrogens were used with medroxyprogesterone acetate. Further studies are required.

Other risk factors for cardiovascular disease

Oestrogen therapy has been recommended as a way of reducing cardiovascular risk in postmenopausal women. There are many other factors, however, that influence a woman's individual risk of developing heart disease. It is important to treat all aspects of a woman's health and not just analyse her hormone or lipid profile. If we are to give full, informed advice, this will mean taking time to assess other factors in relation to diet and lifestyle. There seems little sense in offering a woman HRT if we fail to give advice about other issues that will influence her individual risk of developing cardiovascular problems. Furthermore, some women find it easier to make positive lifestyle changes in an effort to reduce the risk of heart disease but might not be willing to consider HRT. Ideally, we should be encouraging women to consider all influencing factors and how their lifestyle may need to be adjusted accordingly. This advice should include accurate information about the effects of HRT.

Lifestyle factors that increase the risk of cardiovascular disease are:

◆ smoking
◆ obesity
◆ diet
◆ lack of regular exercise
◆ high-fat diet.

Women with certain medical conditions may be at particular risk of cardiovascular disease and it could be argued that they should be targeted to receive information about HRT as well as lifestyle advice (see Chapter 8).

Medical risk factors for cardiovascular disease are:

◆ hypertension
◆ family history of heart disease
◆ diabetes
◆ hypercholesterolaemia.

In the near future we will see the results of long-term trials prospectively evaluating the effect of HRT on the cardiovascular system, and other effects. In the meantime we must advise women according to current medical opinion and ensure that the information we pass on is accurate and up to date.

REFERENCES

Alexandersen P, Toussaint A, Christiansen C et al (2001) Ipriflavone in the treatment of postmenopausal osteoporosis. A randomised controlled trial. *J. Am. Med. Assoc.* **285**(11): 1482–1488.

Baud CA, Very JM, Corvoisier B (1988) Biophysical studies of bone mineral content in biopsies of osteoporosis patients before and after long term treatment with fluoride. *Bone* **9**: 361–365.

Bush TL, Barratt-Connor E, Cowan LD et al (1987) Cardiovascular mortality and non-contraceptive use of oestrogen in women. Results from the Lipid Research Clinics Program Follow-Up Study. *Circulation* **75**: 1102–1109.

Chow R, Harrison JE, Notarius C (1987) Effects of two randomised exercise programmes on bone mass of healthy postmenopausal women. *Br. Med. J.* **295**: 1441–1444.

Christiansen C, Christiansen MS, Transbol I (1981) Bone mass in postmenopausal women after withdrawal of oestrogen replacement therapy. *Lancet* i: 459–461.

Cummings SR, Black DM, Nevitt MC et al (1993) Bone density at various sites for prediction of hip fractures: the study of osteoporosis fractures research group. *Lancet* **341**: 72–75.

Cummings SR, Eckert S, Krenger KA et al (1999) The effect of raloxifene on risk of breast cancer in postmenopausal women. Results from the MORE randomised trial. *J. Am. Med. Assoc.* **281**: 2189–2197.

Dalais FS, Rice GE, Wahlquist ME et al (1998) Effects of dietary phytoestrogens in postmenopausal women. *Climacteric* **1**: 124–129.

Davies GC, Huster WJ, Lu Y et al (1999) Adverse events reported by women in controlled trials with raloxifene. *Obstet. Gynecol.* **93**: 558–565.

Dawson-Hughes B, Dallal GE, Krall EA et al (1991) A controlled trial of the effect of calcium supplementation on bone density in postmenopausal women. *N. Engl. J. Med.* **323**: 878–883.

Dempster D, Shane E, Horbert W, Lindsay R (1986) A simple method for correlative scanning microscopy of human iliac crest biopsies. *Bone Miner.* **1**: 15–21.

Department of Health (1994) *On the State of the Nation.* HMSO, London.

Department of Health (2001) *National Service Framework for Older People.* Department of Health, London.

Drinkwater BL, Nilson K, Chesunt CH et al (1984) Bone mineral content of amenorrheic and eumenorrheic athletes. *N. Engl. J. Med.* **311**: 277.

Ettinger B, Grady D (1994) Maximising the benefit of estrogen therapy for prevention of osteoporosis. *Menopause* **1**: 19–24.

Ettinger B, Genant HK, Cann CE (1985) Long term oestrogen therapy prevents bone loss and fractures. *Ann. Intern. Med.* 102: 319–324,

Ettinger B, Black D, Mitlak BH et al (1999) Reduction of vertebral fracture risk in postmenopausal women with osteoporosis treated with raloxifene: results from a three year randomised controlled trial. *J. Am. Med. Assoc.* 282(7): 637–645.

Falkeborn M, Persson I, Adami HO et al (1992) The risk of acute myocardial infarction after oestrogen and oestrogen/progestogen replacement. *Br. J. Obstet. Gynaecol.* 99: 821–828.

Gennari C, Adami I, Agnusdei D et al (1997) Effect of chronic treatment with ipriflavone in postmenopausal women with low bone mass. *Calcif. Tissue Int.* 61 (Suppl): S19–22.

Gleeson PB, Protas E, LeBlanc A, Schneider VS, Evans HJ (1990). Effects of weight bearing lifting on bone mineral density in premenopausal women. *J. Bone Miner. Res.* 5: 153–158.

Gordon T, Kannel WB, Hjortland MC et al (1978) Menopause and coronary heart disease: The Framingham Study. *Ann. Intern. Med.* 89: 157–161.

Grimley-Evans J (1990) The significance of osteoporosis. In: Smith R (ed.) *Osteoporosis*, pp. 1–8. Royal College of Physicians, London.

Grimley-Evans J, Prudham D, Wardles I (1979) A prospective study of fractured femur, incidence and outcome. *Public Health* 93: 235–241.

Grodstein F, Stampfer M (1995) The epidemiology of coronary heart disease and estrogen replacement in postmenopausal women. *Prog. Cardiovasc. Dis.* 38: 199–210.

Gruber HE, Ivey JC, Baylink DJ et al (1984) Long term calcitonin therapy in postmenopausal osteoporosis. *Metabolism* 33: 295–303.

Hansen M, Overgaard K, Riis B, Christiansen C (1991) Role of peak bone mass and bone loss in postmenopausal osteoporosis. *Br. Med. J.* 303: 961–964.

Henderson BE, Paginini-Hill A, Ross RK (1991) Decreased mortality in users of estrogen replacement therapy. *Arch. Intern. Med.* 151: 75–78.

Henderson VW (1998) Estrogens and the prevalence of Alzheimer's disease. In: Studd JWW (ed.) *The Management of the Menopause, Annual Review*, pp. 183–192. Parthenon, London.

Henderson VW, Watt L, Buckwalter JG (1996) Cognitive skills associated with estrogen therapy in women with Alzheimer's disease. *Psychoneuroendocrinology* 21: 421–430.

Hillard TC, Whitcroft SJ, Marsh MS et al (1994) Long term effects of transdermal and oral hormone replacement therapy on postmenopausal bone loss. *Osteoporosis Int.* 4(6): 341–348.

Hodgson ST, Conrad Johnston C Jr (1996) *Guidelines for the Prevention and Treatment of Postmenopausal Osteoporosis.* American Association of Clinical Endocrinologists, Chicago.

Hully S, Grady D, Bush T et al (1998) Randomised trial of estrogen and progestin for secondary prevention of coronary heart disease in postmenopausal women. *J. Am. Med. Assoc.* 280: 605–612.

Jorm AF, Korten AE, Hendersen AS (1987) The prevelence of dementia: a quantitative integration of the literature. *Acta Psychiatr. Scand.* 76: 467–479.

Kandlers B, Lindsay R, Dempster DW et al (1984) Determinants of bone mass in young healthy women. In: Christiansen C (ed.) *Osteoporosis*, pp. 337–340. Stiftsborgtrykken, Aalborg.

Kanis JA (1994) *Osteoporosis.* Blackwell Scientific, London.
Kanis JA, Gluer CC (2000) An update on the diagnosis and assessment of osteoporosis with densitometry. *Osteoporosis Int.* 11: 192–202.
Kanis JA, Passmore R (1989) Calcium supplementation of the diet. *Br. Med. J.* 298: 137–140.
Lee SJ (2000) *The Sheffield Protocol for the Management of the Menopause and the Prevention of Osteoporosis,* 6th edn. Osteoporosis 2000, Sheffield.
Lindsay RL, Hart DM, Clark DM (1978) Bone response to termination of oestrogen treatment. *Lancet* i: 1325–1327.
Lindsay R, Hart DM, Forrest C, Baird C (1980) Prevention of osteoporosis in oophorectomised women. *Lancet* ii: 1151–1154.
Lobo RA (1991) Effects of hormonal replacement therapy on lipids and lipoproteins in postmenopausal women. *J. Clin. Endocrinol. Metab.* 73: 925–930.
Marx CW, Dailey GE, Cheney C et al (1992) Do estrogens improve bone mineral density in osteoporotic women over age 65? *J. Bone Miner. Res.* 7: 1257–1259.
Melton LJ (1993) Hip fracture – a worldwide problem today and tomorrow. *Bone* 14 (Suppl): 1–8.
Melton LJ III, Chrischilles EA, Cooper C et al (1992) Perspective: how many women have osteoporosis? *J. Bone Miner. Res.* 7(9): 1005–1010.
Nachitgall LE (2001) Isoflavones in the management of the menopause. *J. Br. Menopause Soc.* Suppl 1: 8–12.
Naessen T, Persson I, Adami H et al (1990) Hormone replacement therapy and the risk of hip fracture. *Ann. Intern. Med.* 113: 95–103.
Nair GV, Herrington DM (2001) The ERA trial: findings and implications for the future. *Climacteric* 3: 227–232.
National Osteoporosis Society (1998) Position statement on the use of forearm X-ray absorptiometry. National Osteoporosis Society, Bath.
Paginini-Hill A, Henderson VW (1996) Estrogen replacement therapy and risk of Alzheimer's disease. *Arch. Intern. Med.* 156: 2213–2217.
PEPI Trial (1995) Effects of estrogen or estrogen plus progestin regimens on heart disease risk factors in postmenopausal women. The Postmenopausal Estrogen/Progestin Intervention Trial. *J. Am. Med. Assoc.* 273: 199–208.
Richelson LS, Wahner HW, Melton LJ, Riggs BL (1984) Relative contributions of ageing and oestrogen deficiency to postmenopausal bone loss. *N. Engl. J. Med.* 311: 1273–1275.
Riggs BL, Wahner HW, Seeman E et al (1982) Changes in bone mineral density of the proximal femur and spine with ageing. Differences between the postmenopausal and senile osteoporosis syndromes. *J. Clin. Invest.* 70: 716–723.
Riggs BL, Baylink DJ, Kleerekoper M et al (1987) Incidence of hip fracture in osteoporotic women; treatment with sodium flouride. *J. Bone Miner. Res.* 2: 123–126.
Rosenberg L, Hennekens CH, Rosner B et al (1981) Early menopause and the risk of myocardial infarction. *Am. J. Obstet. Gynecol.* 139: 47–51.
Ross R (1999) Athersclorosis – an inflammatory disease. *N. Engl. J. Med.* 340: 115–126.
Sato M, Glasebrook AL, Bryant HU (1994) Raloxifene: a selective estrogen receptor modulator. *J. Bone Miner. Metab.* 12(Suppl 2): 519–520.

Smolders RGV, Van der Mooren MJ (2000) New emerging risk factors for cardiovascular disease: their relation with menopause and hormone therapy. *J. Br. Menopause Soc.* **6**(1): 27–33.

Stampfer MJ, Colditz GA (1991) Oestrogen replacement therapy and coronary heart disease: a quantitative assessment of the epidemiological evidence. *Prev. Med.* **20**: 47–63.

Stampfer MJ, Willet WC, Colditz GA et al (1985) A prospective study of postmenopausal estrogen therapy and coronary heart disease. *N. Engl. J. Med.* **313**: 1044–1049.

Steiniche T, Hasling C, Charles P et al (1989) A randomised study on the effects of oestrogen/gestagen or high dose oral calcium on trabecular bone remodelling in postmenopausal osteoporosis. *Bone* **10**: 313–320.

Stepan IJ, Pospichal J, Presl J et al (1987) Bone loss and biochemical indices of bone remodelling in surgically induced postmenopausal women. *Bone* **8**: 279–284.

Stevenson JC, Marsh MS (1992) *An Atlas of Osteoporosis.* Encyclopaedia of Visual Medicine Series. Parthenon, Carnforth.

Stevenson JC, Lees B, Devonport M et al (1989) Determinants of bone density in normal women: risk factors for future fracture. *Br. Med. J.* **298**: 924–928.

Stevenson JC, Cust MP, Gangar KF et al (1990) Effects of transdermal versus oral HRT on bone mineral density in spine and proximal femur in postmenopausal women. *Lancet* **335**: 265–269.

Stewart A, Torgerson DJ, Reid DM (1996) Prediction of fracture in perimenopausal women: a comparison of dual energy X ray absorptiometry and ultrasound attenuation. *Ann. Rheum. Dis.* **55**: 140–142.

Webb CM, Hayward CS, Collins P (2000) Changes in coronary arteries with estrogen therapy. In: Studd JWW (ed.) *Management of the Menopause, Millenium Review,* pp. 153–164. Parthenon, London.

Woolfe AD, St John Dixon A (1998) *Osteoporosis: A Clinical Guide.* Martin Dunitz, London.

World Health Organization (1994) Assessment of osteoporosis fracture risk and its role in screening for postmenopausal osteoporosis. Technical Report Series. WHO, Geneva.

4

Premature Ovarian Failure

It is most common for the menopause to occur naturally during the late forties or early fifties. Some women, however, experience the menopause at a much earlier age – even as young as the late teens or twenties. When the menopause occurs before the age of 40 years, it may be described as **premature**.

Primary ovarian failure occurs when the woman fails to menstruate at all and endocrinological tests reveal ovarian failure. Such women may be very young when the diagnosis is made, and it is often associated with genetic disorder.

Secondary ovarian failure arises when a woman has menstruated normally but subsequently experiences amenorrhoea as a result of ovarian failure.

The consequences of an early menopause are greater than with a so-called 'normal' menopause, and most specialists would agree that not only do such women deserve particular medical attention but they also require a great deal of psychological and emotional support. Society expects women of a certain age to be approaching the 'change of life' and women themselves are mentally prepared for the inevitable. When the ovaries cease to function at a younger age, for whatever reason, or if they are surgically removed, women may feel cheated – that their bodies have let them down and even that they are losing their femininity.

Health professionals working in the field of menopause should ensure that these women receive adequate medical attention as well as emotional help and support. This chapter defines premature menopause, its causes and effects, and discusses the medical management of women experiencing an early menopause. It also outlines some of the emotional and psychological issues that women may need help to deal with at this time.

DEFINITION

Premature ovarian failure is a syndrome occurring before the age of 40 years, characterized by primary or secondary amenorrhoea, raised gonadotrophin levels and low oestrogen levels (Anasti 1998). Bilateral oophorectomy will also result in a sudden early menopause.

Potential consequences of an early menopause are:

◆ vasomotor symptoms
◆ psychological symptoms
◆ sexual problems
◆ infertility
◆ osteoporosis
◆ arterial disease.

INCIDENCE

It is difficult to assess the true incidence of early menopause as it is likely that many women with the condition are not actually diagnosed. Premature ovarian failure accounts for 2–10% of women with primary or secondary amenorrhoea, and it is estimated that 1–3% of the general female population is affected (Anasti 1998).

CAUSES

◆ Surgery
◆ Iatrogenic
◆ Natural or spontaneous.

Surgery

The most obvious cause of early menopause is removal of the ovaries. Ovaries are usually removed only in the presence of disease, but when they are both removed menopause is induced. Symptoms may occur within a very short space of time if hormone replacement therapy (HRT) is not prescribed. Long-term HRT will be necessary for protection of the skeletal and cardiovascular systems. Women who undergo early menopause as a result of surgery are at particular risk of osteoporosis and heart disease, if left untreated (Colditz et al 1987).

Hysterectomy alone, with conservation of ovaries, may also bring forward the expected date of menopause (Siddle et al 1987), although this is not conclusive (Rind et al 1995). Many women expect that one remaining ovary will continue to function as normal until the expected date of menopause and are often not warned that the menopause may occur earlier. Such women may ignore any symptoms suggestive of the menopause or be dismissed as being 'too young'. Asymptomatic women may not receive HRT, which could be necessary if the menopause occurs early. Some specialists recommend periodic measurements of follicle stimulating hormone (FSH) to establish onset of menopause in such women (Seeley 1992).

Iatrogenic

Ovarian failure can be caused by external factors such as:

◆ radiotherapy
◆ chemotherapy.

Radiotherapy

The risk of ovarian failure as a result of radiotherapy depends on the age of the individual, the dose of radiation and the duration of treatment (Seeley & Ashton 2000). Shielding the ovaries reduces the amount of radiation reaching them.

Chemotherapy

Chemotherapeutic agents have an adverse effect on ovarian function in most women. Women aged over 30 years at the time of the chemotherapy are likely to experience permanent ovarian failure, and young women are at risk of an earlier menopause, but several years later (Howell et al 1998).

Natural or spontaneous causes

Sometimes the ovaries fail spontaneously, or naturally, but at an unusually early age. Women may present with typical menopausal symptoms or they may be asymptomatic. Diagnosis of premature ovarian failure may result from investigations into a separate condition, such as infertility or prolonged amenorrhoea. In such instances an unexpected diagnosis of early menopause is traumatic.

A true cause for early menopause is often never discovered, but in some women the following may be contributory:

◆ genetic factors
◆ autoimmune disease
◆ infection.

Genetic factors

The majority of women with early menopause have a normal 46XX karyotype (Alper & Garner 1985), but some women show an abnormality on a specific part of the X chromosome. This is demonstrated by a familial link in some cases (Partington et al 1996). In Turner's syndrome (45X0), ovaries develop normally in utero, but accelerated follicular atresia causes ovarian failure (Devi & Benn 1999).

Autoimmune disease

Some women with premature ovarian failure have a history of autoimmune disease, such as Addison's disease, diabetes mellitus and hypothyroidism (Anasti 1998).

Infection

Infections with the mumps virus can cause damage to the ovaries, although ovarian function may return spontaneously (Morrison et al 1991).

Ovarian dysfunction

Occasionally, after an apparent premature menopause, ovarian function may return spontaneously (Seeley & Ashton 2000). This may be described as **premature ovarian dysfunction** or **resistant ovary syndrome**, and may be an early indicator of permanent cessation of ovarian activity. Pregnancy may occur, even with relatively raised FSH levels, so relevant contraceptive advice is essential (Seeley & Ashton 2000).

CLINICAL ASSESSMENT

It is essential that women suspected of premature ovarian failure be assessed comprehensibly. The diagnosis, once made, may be traumatic for many women, and will have implications with regard to fertility, feelings of femininity and physical effects. As well as a full physical examination and treatment, **strong psychological support** is essential.

Diagnosis

A diagnosis of premature ovarian failure is considered in women with a history of amenorrhoea, who may or may not be experiencing menopause-type symptoms. Measurement of FSH levels is performed serially on at least two occasions. A persistently raised FSH concentration cannot be considered as absolute evidence of ovarian failure, because studies have shown that a few women with levels above 40 IU/L have ovulated and even become pregnant (Rebar et al 1982); however, this is extremely rare. Chromosome analysis should be considered in women under 35 years of age (Anasti 1998). In the case of primary amenorrhoea, pelvic ultrasonography is usually undertaken (Kalentardou et al 1998).

Opinion is divided as to whether ovarian biopsies are of clinical value. A biopsy will differentiate between premature ovarian failure (when no follicles are identified) and resistant ovary syndrome (where immature follicles may be seen). However, clinical management is unlikely to change. There are also the risks associated with general anaesthesia, surgery and postoperative recovery. Postoperative adhesions may also occur, hindering any efforts at assisted conception at a later date.

The diagnosis of premature menopause is always traumatic and may follow several months of clinical investigation. Referral to a specialist centre is advisable so that the necessary tests, investigations and counselling can be carried out as promptly as possible.

TREATMENT

In view of the increased risk of both osteoporosis and heart disease in women with premature ovarian failure, it is essential that they receive adequate oestrogen replacement, combined with progestogen when required (Anasti 1998). For most women this will mean long-term HRT. It is important that each woman is given the information she needs to decide with her doctor which particular form of HRT she will take. HRT will be recommended until at least the normal age of the menopause.

Women who do not wish to become pregnant should be warned of the very small theoretical risk of pregnancy and advised on suitable contraceptive methods. The combined oral contraceptive may be the treatment of choice in suitable women. Women who do desire pregnancy will need extensive fertility investigations and counselling, with a view to attempted induction of ovulation or ovum donation.

PSYCHOLOGICAL SUPPORT

It can be very traumatic for a woman to be told that she is unexpectedly menopausal, particularly if she has yet to have children. It comes as a shock to learn that the ovaries have ceased to function and that se rious health consequences are possible, if treatment is not considered.

Women often remember vividly the occasion on which they were given the diagnosis of ovarian failure, so it is vital that such information is imparted as sympathetically as possible. Women speak of being told very abruptly, in busy gynaecological clinics, with little time for discussion or questions. Many women leave the clinic upset, confused, and feeling very isolated. They seldom know anyone else with the condition and often do not know where to turn. Blood tests may be performed on several occasions but still the woman is sometimes left feeling unprepared and anxious about the possible diagnosis. At such times any information that is given may not be taken in and remembered.

Support groups are commonly held for women undergoing hysterectomy; women having surgical removal of the ovaries may find help in these groups. Women experiencing spontaneous ovarian failure are often left isolated and anxious. Partners, parents and friends may not be able to offer much help and, even from health professionals, there may be little in the way of counselling or psychological support.

In some areas local support groups have been established. The needs of the group will vary according to the ages of the women and whether or not they have had children. Women who have completed their families may still experience feelings of grief when confronted with sterility. Women have expressed that the following issues cause anxiety and that opportunity for discussion of them would be helpful:

◆ fertility
◆ sexuality
◆ ageing
◆ telling partners and family
◆ medical and health consequences, including symptom relief.

FERTILITY

Although pregnancies have occurred in women who have been diagnosed with ovarian failure, they are rare, and most women wanting children will need extensive fertility management. If reversible ovarian dysfunction is suspected, ovulation induction can be attempted. Otherwise the options are:

◆ in vitro fertilization using ovum donation
◆ embryo transfer using ovum donation
◆ gamete intrafallopian transfer (GIFT) using ovum donation
◆ adoption.

In conclusion, the impact of a diagnosis of premature ovarian failure is often underestimated. There is little available in the way of information leaflets, books and videos about the subject. The majority of booklets about menopause assume an age of around 50 years and for the younger woman they are inappropriate. Each woman should, therefore, be treated individually with as much attention being paid to her non-physical health as to the physical. At present, some women are not even given the information they need to look after their physical health after an early menopause, let alone the psyche and emotions.

REFERENCES

Alper MM, Garner PR (1985) Premature ovarian failure: its relationship to autoimmune disease. *Obstet. Gynecol.* **66**: 27.

Anasti JN (1998) Premature ovarian failure: an update. *Fertil. Steril.* **70**: 1–15.

Colditz GA, Willett WC, Stampfer MJ et al (1987) Menopause and the risk of coronary heart disease in women. *N. Engl. J. Med.* **316**: 1105.

Devi A, Benn PA (1999) X chromosome abnormalities in women with premature ovarian failure. *J. Reprod. Med.* **44**: 321–324.

Howell SJ, Berger G, Adams JE, Shalet SM (1998) Bone mineral density in women with cytotoxic induced ovarian failure. *Clin. Endocrinol.* **49**: 397–402.

Kalentardou SN, Davis SR, Nelson LM (1998) Premature ovarian failure. *Endocrinol. Metab. Clin. North Am.* **27**: 989–1000.

Morrison JC, Gimes JR, Wiser LW et al (1991) Mumps oophritis: a cause of premature menopause. *Fertil. Steril.* **26**: 255.

Partington MW, Moore DY, Turner GM (1996) Confirmation of early menopause in fragile X carriers. *Am. J. Med. Genet.* **64**: 370–372.

Rebar RW, Erickson GF, Yen SSC (1982) Idiopathic premature ovarian failure: clinical and endocrine characteristics. *Fertil. Steril.* **37**: 35.

Rind P, Lind C, Nilas L (1995) Lack of influence of simple premenopausal hysterectomy on bone mass and bone metabolism. *Am. J. Obstet. Gynecol.* **172**: 891–895.

Seeley T (1992) Oestrogen replacement therapy after hysterectomy. *Br. Med. J.* **305**: 811–812.

Seeley T, Ashton S (2000) Premature ovarian failure: a practical approach. *J. Br. Menopause Soc.* **6**(3): 107–109.

Siddle N, Sarrel P, Whitehead MI (1987) The effects of hysterectomy on the age of ovarian failure: identification of a subgroup of women with premature loss of ovarian function and literature review. *Fertil. Steril.* **47**: 94–100.

5

Women's Perspectives on the Menopause

The only consistent factor in every woman's experience of the menopause is that eventually menstruation stops. Other than this, you can help to prepare a woman for the onset of menopause, explaining what might happen and how she may feel, but you cannot say for certain how she *will* feel. Every woman's experience of the climacteric period is unique – her life will be influenced by many factors other than just hormonal ones. Her expectations of the menopause and related symptoms, her life experiences, her culture and her circumstances will all influence her perception and experience of the climacteric.

CHANGING TIMES

Attitudes to the menopause have changed over the years, particularly as society itself has changed. In the Victorian era the word menopause would hardly have been mentioned as being of medical concern, except perhaps to recognize that it sometimes resulted in women having a 'nervous disposition'. Women themselves would have welcomed it as a release from childbearing. In the early to mid twentieth century, the menopause was viewed as a time of loss or decay. Women were often prescribed tranquillizers or antidepressants, showing that the climacteric was viewed as a time of distress. Now, in the twenty-first century, the menopause is sometimes viewed as a deficiency disease that needs to be 'treated', particularly by the medical profession who tend to have 'medicalized' the menopause in some respects. Women may feel that they are less feminine after the menopause, or less healthy, if they decline the offered hormone replacement therapy (HRT). Yet women are anxious about the use of HRT and want to be sure that it is really safe and appropriate before they consider its use.

In recent years stereotypes have started to be recast: women are no longer considered 'over the hill' at 50, but rather may experience what has been termed a 'post-menopausal zest' (Sheehy, 1993).

'If 45 is the old age of youth, 50 is the youth of a woman's second adulthood' (Gail Sheehy, 1993, p. 19)

The menopause is no longer seen as a sickness but as a 'transition phase' into a new life. Women are seeking information on the subject of menopause and want to decide for themselves whether or not to take HRT. The media play an important role in informing women about the menopause and HRT. This has both positive and negative implications for women's knowledge about the subject. One thing is certain, however: women no longer consider the menopause as a taboo subject – they actively seek the information they need to be informed. Armed with the facts, gleaned from women's magazines, radio chat shows and television documentaries, they resent medics trying to make the decision for them about HRT. Women want to be accurately informed and actively involved in the decision as to whether to take HRT. They are also turning to alternative means of alleviating menopausal symptoms using complementary or non-hormonal therapies. The modern challenge to women is to 'know your own menopause' or, as Gail Sheehy puts it in her book, *The Silent Passage*, 'claim the pause'.

CHANGING CULTURES

The menopause is inevitable for women who live long enough, but how it is experienced is unique to individuals. Even purely physiological symptoms such as hot flushes, sweats and vaginal dryness are not universally experienced, or at least acknowledged, by all cultures. Lock (1991), studying Japanese women, and Wright (1983) studying Navaho Indians, found that in each of these cultures there are no words for 'hot flush'. Symptom reporting in Japan is significantly lower than in women from North America (Lock 1994). Lock reminds us, though, that, when considered alongside Japan's low incidence of heart disease, breast cancer and its high life expectancy it is possible that biological factors as well as psychological ones will influence their experience of menopausal symptoms.

For some African women the time of menopause indicates a higher social status, and life becomes easier after it. This means that the menopause is seen as a positive life event, whereas in countries such as the USA, Germany and Italy, it is viewed in a negative way – as a demarcation of ageing (Flint 1994). This may influence how a woman feels at the time of the menopause.

In China, few women seek advice about the menopause, although it is possible that they do experience symptoms, but suffer in silence. Chinese women generally perceive the menopause as a natural process and so perhaps have a positive attitude towards any symptoms they may experience (Tang 1994).

In the UK, cultural differences are less profound but still important, particularly with regard to the use of HRT. The following factors are worth considering:

◆ Catholic women may associate HRT with the contraceptive pill and refuse it because of religious objections. Careful counselling on the differences between HRT and the contraceptive pill is required.

◆ Orthodox Jews or Muslim women may not wish to resume bleeding again after the menopause because of religious restrictions during menstruation. HRT regimens that achieve amenorrhoea may be acceptable.

◆ Vegetarians or vegans may be keen to know whether their HRT is derived directly from animals. Alternatives, derived from plants, may be preferred.

CHANGING PRESSURES

The climacteric is a time in a woman's life of great physical change, which may last for months or even years. For the average woman, these hormonal changes will occur at around the age of 50 years, when she may also be experiencing pressures in other areas of her life. All of these other factors may influence how a woman feels and also how she copes with any menopausal symptoms that may occur. Long-standing problems may become harder to live with or to deal with when a woman is also experiencing physical or psychological upset as a result of hormonal changes. Every woman approaching the menopause has a variety of needs, not just hormonal ones, so it is important to take a holistic approach and consider all aspects of a woman's life, not simply her hormones.

'It's your age'

There is a tendency to blame the menopause for every upset or complaint that arises around this time of a woman's life. Anxiety, depression and panic attacks may all be labelled as being menopausal symptoms and for some women it can be hard to simply find a listening ear. Certainly the menopause cannot be blamed for every emotional upset, although some problems may be exacerbated by hormonal influences, causing long-standing problems to be highlighted or new ones to be recognized.

Factors that may affect a woman's attitudes to the menopause include:

◆ changing body image
◆ ageing
◆ attitudes towards sexuality
◆ dreams and expectations
◆ relationships
◆ 'empty nest' syndrome
◆ roles and responsibilities.

Changing body image

The media would have us believe that all women must be slim to be beautiful. Society strives towards maintaining a youthful figure into middle age and beyond. Large sums of money are spent by women trying to lose weight and keep young-looking. Yet it is a fact of life that, as we get older, our bodies do change and unless we can afford plastic surgery it is inevitable that we will begin to 'show our age'. Wrinkles may appear, hair often greys, waistlines thicken and muscles sag, particularly if underused. Both men and women have to learn to accept their changing bodies and yet still look after them. HRT is not a youth drug and will not prevent many of the effects of ageing on the body. Exercise, diet and lifestyle are probably more important factors (see Ch. 8). Women who turn to HRT hoping to 'turn back the clock' will be sadly disappointed.

Ageing

The menopause is an event that most women cannot ignore. Some women see the menopause as marking the beginning of new freedom, new choices and new challenges. For others it represents a turning point, a stage in life one step nearer to old age and, ultimately, death. Attitudes to ageing vary, but for some women, the menopause may be an uncomfortable reminder of one's lost youth and vigour. For women who struggle with acute menopausal symptoms, the perimenopausal phase may be a difficult one to come to terms with, as they wonder how long these symptoms really will continue. An understanding of a woman's perspective will help when trying to counsel or advise a woman at this time.

Sexuality

The menopause marks the end of the fertile years. Contraception can (eventually) be stopped and sexual intercourse continued without concern about pregnancy. For some, this is a release, for others a sadness, perhaps highlighting the ageing process. A woman may feel less desirable or less attractive to her partner. This, along with physical effects such as vaginal dryness or reduced libido, may lead to sexual difficulties at this time. Sensitive counselling, practical advice, HRT if appropriate and sometimes psychosexual therapy will be of benefit.

Dreams and expectations

Some women look upon the menopause as a life event, a stage in life to be recognized and coped with, either in a positive way or negatively. It may be a time of evaluation of past life or of planning for a future one. Women may look back with regret because of failed dreams or sad memories. For childless women, the menopause, marking the end of the reproductive era, may be particularly poignant.

For working women, success may not be as great as one had hoped, promotion may be out of reach and retirement becomes the next major step. Marriages and relationships may come under scrutiny, particularly as children leave home and women are given more time to evaluate their own lives. Expectations of life may not be fulfilled, the partner may be going through similar 'mid-life' thoughts and decisions. Some women may feel as though the menopause is simply highlighting negative aspects of life, rather than signifying a time of new beginnings and expectations. Helping a woman to understand both the negatives and the positives of middle age may help her to deal more easily with the hormonal effects of the menopause.

Relationships

Mid life can be a time when relationships are tested or re-evaluated. Marriages may be faltering and need a concerted effort to revive them. Physical and psychological effects of the menopause can test a stable, loving relationship, yet alone one that is faltering. Men, too, may be experiencing difficulties, as they come to terms with approaching middle age. Men do not experience a true hormonal change in the same way as women do, but they undoubtedly have to face similar issues regarding health, work and sexuality. Couples may seek help in making adjustments to changing roles and changing lives. For some couples, relationship counselling may be of benefit.

'Empty nest' syndrome

The so-called 'empty nest' syndrome is used to describe the feelings of sadness and emptiness that a woman may experience when her last child leaves home. A woman who has dedicated her whole life to the upbringing of her children may struggle with the new role she finds herself in – as an independent woman and/or partner. In these days, when many women work outside the home and are encouraged to pursue personal interests as well as those of their family, these feelings may be less intense.

Roles and responsibilities

Mid life may be viewed as a time of increased freedom: children leave home, finances may be more secure, work life may be settled. It can come as a shock to some to realize that, just as they are losing the dependence of their children, their own parents may be becoming more dependent on them. Women may find themselves torn between caring for their parents and remaining loyal to their partner. For some, this may cause feelings of resentment and frustration, leading to guilt when the elderly parent does die. Counselling may be of help in these circumstances.

Some women also struggle with the changing roles from mother to grandmother, as their own children have families of their own. However, the role of grandparent can be immensely satisfying and rewarding.

Work relationships may change. For most women, menopausal symptoms are not usually severe enough to require more than simple adaptations to the working life, such as opening more windows, wearing layers of clothes and keeping a notebook for those forgotten messages! However, women who lose their job during mid life, for whatever reason, may find it very difficult to get back into the workplace. A woman may find that her husband is reaching the peak of his career, with all its satisfaction and achievements, just at the point that she feels unsettled in work or poorly motivated, because of climacteric symptoms.

When advising a woman about the menopause and HRT, try to find out what other factors – social, emotional or physical – may be affecting how she feels. Helping her to cope with some of these other difficulties may make it easier for her to cope with the menopause. Alternatively, helping her through the hormonal upset of the menopause may make her more able to cope with other problems by herself.

CONTRACEPTION AT THE PERIMENOPAUSE

The menopause marks the end of a woman's reproductive life, but can be recognized as such only retrospectively. Menstruation may occur after several months of amenorrhoea, when a woman believed herself to be infertile. Fertility declines appreciably once a women is in her forties (Stovall et al 1991) and frequency of intercourse lessens in some instances (Wadsworth 1995). Pregnancy is therefore unusual but not impossible. The *Guinness Book of Records* shows the oldest woman to have given birth following spontaneous conception as 57 years and 129 days old!

It has been suggested that women over the age of 35 years have more serious adverse pregnancy outcomes than younger women. Preeclampsia, gestational diabetes, induction of labour and caesarian section are more prevalent after this age (Bobrowski & Bottoms 1995). With increased obstetrical monitoring, however, the mortality rate may be no different to that in younger women (Spellacy et al 1985). Women over the age 40 years are, however, more likely to have termination of pregnancy: 40% of all pregnancies in women over 40 ended in termination in 1995 (Office of Population Censuses and Surveys 1997).

There is also a greater risk of a baby being born with congenital abnormalities such as Down's syndrome. Along with the physical problems associated with a pregnancy at this time, psychological and emotional difficulties may accompany what is often an unwanted pregnancy.

It is therefore crucial that women are warned of the continuing need for contraception during the perimenopause. Many women wrongly believe that they are infertile during this time or 'take a chance' that they will not be the one to fall pregnant.

For how long is contraception necessary?

The Family Planning Association recommendations are that women under the age of 50 years should continue using contraception until they have experienced 2 years of amenorrhoea. Over the age of 50, women should continue using contraception for at least 1 year after their last period. For women not on HRT, these recommendations are simple, if a little tedious. Women may feel that one of the few advantages of the menopause is that contraception becomes (eventually) unnecessary. To have to continue using contraception for 12–24 months can seem an unnecessary precaution, but most women do not want to run the risk of pregnancy.

Once a perimenopausal woman starts on HRT, it becomes much more difficult to advise about when to stop using contraception. Bleeding may continue with the use of HRT and, even if amenorrhoea occurs, a woman cannot assume that she is infertile. Theoretically, you could ask a woman to stop HRT and measure levels of follicle stimulating hormone (FSH) 6–8 weeks later. If levels are raised and accompanied by amenorrhoea, this would indicate menopause. Contraception should then be used for one more year.

It is therefore impossible to give absolute recommendations about when a woman on HRT can stop using contraception. In practice, an arbitrary figure of around 55 years is suggested, although it should be stressed to women that this is only a guide. Each woman will make her own decision based on her perception and acceptance of risk, which will be influenced by the following:

◆ age
◆ frequency of coitus
◆ how easily she previously became pregnant
◆ male fertility (younger men may be more fertile)
◆ acceptability of methods of contraception.

Combined oral contraception

The combined contraceptive pill can be used by a woman during the perimenopausal phase provided the following criteria are met:

◆ she is a non-smoker
◆ she is normotensive
◆ she is not obese
◆ she has no family history of cardiovascular disease and no cardiovascular risk factors, including venous thrombosis.

Combined oral contraception increases the risk of venous thrombosis. Advising women which combined preparation to take and weighing up potential benefit against thromboembolic risk is becoming more complex. Some studies have shown an increased risk with third-generation progestogens compared with second-generation oral contraceptives (Rosing et al 1997, Spitzer et al 1996). It has been suggested that, based on current understanding, second-generation preparations are probably best for healthy, low-risk, older women (Gebbie 1998).

Women must be involved in a frank discussion regarding the risks and benefits of continuing use of the combined pill until the time of the menopause.

Effect on the menopause

Use of the combined pill will cause menopausal symptoms to be masked, as oestrogen levels remain high as a result of the pill. The oestrogen also offers protection against osteoporosis. The exact time of the last period will not be known, as regular withdrawal bleeds are likely to continue.

The progestogen-only pill

The progestogen-only pill (POP) or 'mini pill' can be taken safely during the perimenopause. It works in the following ways:

◆ changes quality of cervical mucus
◆ renders the endometrium unreceptive to a fertilized oocyte so implantation cannot occur
◆ affects the mobility of the fallopian tubes, preventing spermatozoa from travelling to meet an ovum.

Although the rate of pregnancy in women using the POP is often quoted as 1–4 pregnancies per 100 woman-years, the rate among older women users is the most favourable (Vessey et al 1990).

Effect on the menopause

Use of the POP will not usually mask the onset of menopausal symptoms. Amenorrhoea may occur with the use of the POP and women may wonder whether the menopause has occurred. If a woman does experience prolonged amenorrhoea on the POP, she cannot assume she is becoming postmenopausal. Serial FSH measurements are not affected by the use of the POP.

Injectable and implanted progestogens

One of the main drawbacks of these methods, when considering use in perimenopausal women, is the fact that they are long lasting. Most women at this time are looking for contraception that is convenient to use, but also easy to stop after the menopause. Injectable and implanted progestogens are extremely reliable forms of contraception but can cause irregular bleeding and side-effects such as weight gain and mood swings. It would be difficult to consider the use of HRT alongside such methods, because of the risk of irregular bleeding. Concerns have been expressed that long-term use of injectable progestogens may be associated with low oestrogen levels and loss of bone mineral density in premenopausal women (Cundy et al 1991). This issue is unresolved and it is suggested that women with amenorrhoea of longer than 5 years' duration should be monitored, by measuring oestradiol levels, particularly in the presence of other risk factors for osteoporosis. 'Add back' HRT can be given in conjunction with the progestogen or the woman could be advised to consider alternative methods of contraception (Gebbie 1998).

Intrauterine systems (IUSs)

Modern IUSs offer a very satisfactory form of contraception for women approaching the menopause. They are long lasting and have few side-effects. A copper device inserted at the age of 40 years is unlikely to be replaced unless the woman experiences problems. Copper devices will be left in situ and removed after the menopause (Gebbie 1998). The woman then has adequate contraceptive cover throughout the perimenopausal era.

An IUS containing levonorgestrel combines the benefits of both hormonal and intrauterine contraception (Fig. 5.1). It has a central

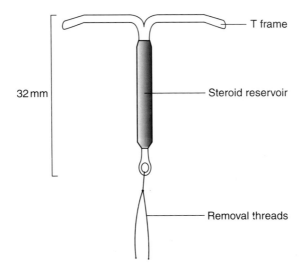

Figure 5.1 Levonorgestrel-releasing intrauterine system.

reservoir which contains 52 mg of levonorgestrel, released at a steady 20 μg per 24 hours. It is as effective as female sterilization and has a lower risk of ectopic pregnancy (Gebbie 1998). Unlike other intrauterine devices, the levonorgestrel system confers positive health benefits and is associated with a dramatic reduction in menstrual blood loss (Anderson & Rybo 1990). Irregular bleeding is common in the first 3–6 months, often settling to amenorrhoea. This system is licensed for contraceptive use in the UK, but could also be used in conjunction with oestrogen as a form of HRT (Anderson et al 1992, Raudaskoski et al 1995).

Barrier methods

- ◆ Condom – male and female
- ◆ Diaphragm
- ◆ Spermicidal pessaries
- ◆ Spermicidal foam.

Barrier methods of contraception are commonly used by women around the time of the menopause. They have no effect on hormonal changes and so do not influence the onset of menopause or mask symptoms at this time. They are easily stopped when contraception is no longer required.

Learning how to use a method such as a condom or cap can be difficult for a woman who has never used this method before, particularly if she is beginning to suffer vaginal dryness as a result of oestrogen deficiency. However, a couple who are used to such methods may find them convenient to continue through the climacteric years.

The decline in fertility in the year leading up to the time of the menopause means that methods that might be considered unreliable for younger women probably offer sufficient contraceptive protection to perimenopausal women. This includes the use of spermicidal agents on their own.

The spread of human immunodeficiency virus (HIV) and the subsequent health awareness campaigns have resulted in barrier methods becoming more popular, particularly with younger women who have grown up with the 'AIDS message'. With an increasing number of women entering new relationships later in life, it could be argued that so-called 'safe sex' should be practised at all ages, including the perimenopause and beyond.

Sterilization

It has been estimated that 40% of women aged 40–45 years report that one or other partner has been sterilized (Gebbie et al 1995). This obviously takes care of the problem of contraception through the perimenopausal years. It is unlikely that sterilization would be considered by a woman who was close to menopause; she is likely to be advised to use an alternative method until she achieves natural sterility.

Natural methods

A 'natural' approach to contraception appeals to many women. Sexual intercourse is avoided during the fertile time of the cycle, which is recognized by one or more of the following factors:

◆ changes in the cervix
◆ changes in cervical mucous secretions
◆ basal body temperature
◆ calendar method.

The perimenopause would be a difficult time to learn such methods, because of a woman's changing body at this time. However, a woman who is familiar with the method and is aware of changes in her body may be able to rely on the method throughout the perimenopause. The 'Persona' monitor is a hand-held device that measures concentrations of the hormones oestrone and luteinizing hormone in urine. The computerized unit analyses the women's cycle and predicts fertile phases. This is unlikely to be accurate during times of hormonal fluctuation such as the perimenopause.

Postcoital or 'emergency' contraception

The combined oestrogen pill regimen can be used safely by peri-menopausal women if there are no contraindications to the general use of oestrogen (Harper 1995). If the risk of pregnancy is considered to be high, but the women is unable to take oestrogen therapy, insertion of an IUS may be considered.

HRT and contraception

Many women start HRT before their periods actually stop, for relief of menopausal symptoms. It becomes impossible to be sure when exactly a woman stops being fertile as the occurrence of the menopause itself is masked. Conventional doses of any HRT cannot be relied on for contraception, and some perimenopausal women on HRT still ovulate (Gebbie et al 1995). Barrier methods and intrauterine devices may be used in conjunction with HRT (Gebbie et al 1995). There are no data to confirm the efficacy of the progestogen-only pill with HRT use, but it is used widely in this way (Gebbie 1998).

REFERENCES

Anderson K, Rybo G (1990) Levonorgestrel releasing intrauterine device in the treatment of menorrhagia. *Br. J. Obstet. Gynaecol.* **97**: 690–694.

Anderson K, Matteson LA, Rybo G et al (1992) Intrauterine release of levonorgestrel – a new way of adding progestogen in hormone replacement therapy. *Obstet. Gynecol.* **79**: 963–967.

Bobrowski RA, Bottoms SF (1995) Underappreciated risks of the elderly multipara. *Am. J. Obstet. Gynecol.* **172**: 1764–1767.

Cundy T, Evans M, Roberts H et al (1991) Bone density in women receiving depot medroxyprogesterone acetate for contraception. *Br. Med. J.* **30**: 13–16.

Flint M (1994) Menopause – the global aspect. In: *The Modern Management of the Menopause.* Proceedings of the VIIth International Congress on Menopause, Stockholm, Sweden, 1993, pp. 17–22. Parthenon, Carnforth.

Gebbie A (1998) Contraception for women over 40 years. In: Studd JW (ed.) *Management of the Menopause, Annual Review,* pp. 67–80. Parthenon, London.

Gebbie AE, Glasier A, Sweeney V (1995) Incidence of ovulation in perimenopausal women before and during HRT. *Contraception* **52**: 221–222.

Harper C (1995) Contraception in the perimenopause. In: Bromham D (ed.) *Contraception.* Reed Healthcare Communications, Sutton, UK.

Lock M (1991) Contested meanings of the menopause. *Lancet* **337**: 1270–1272.

Lock M (1994) Menopause in a cultural setting. *Exp. Gerontol.* **29**(3–4): 307–317.

Office of Population Censuses and Surveys (1997) *Population Trends*, Vol. 87, p. 17. OPCS, London.

Raudaskoski TH, Lahti EI, Kauppila AJ et al (1995) Transdermal estrogen with a levonorgestrel releasing IUD for climacteric complaints: clinical and endometrial responses. *Am. J. Obstet. Gynecol.* **172**: 114–119.

Rosing J, Tans G, Nickolaes AF (1997) Oral contraception and venous thrombosis: different sensitivities to activated protein C in women using second or third generation oral contraception. *Br. J. Haematol.* **97**: 233–238.

Sheehy G (1993) *The Silent Passage*. Harper Collins, London.

Spellacy WN, Miller SL, Winegar A (1985) Pregnancy over 40 years of age. *Gynaecology* **83**: 452–454.

Spitzer WO, Lewis M, Heinemann LAJ et al (1996) Third generation oral contraceptives and risk of thromboembolic disorders: an international case control study. *Br. Med. J.* **312**: 83–88.

Stovall DW, Toma SK, Hammond M (1991) The effect of age on female fecundity. *Obstet. Gynecol.* **77**: 33–36.

Tang G (1994) Menopause – the situation in Hong Kong Chinese women. In: *The Modern Management of the Menopause*. Proceedings of the VIIth International Congress on Menopause, Stockholm, Sweden, 1993, pp. 47–56. Parthenon, Carnforth.

Vessey MP, Villard-Mackintosh L, Yeates D (1990) Effectiveness of progestogen only oral contraceptives (letter). *Br. J. Family Planning* **16**: 79.

Wadwsorth J (1995) Sexual health for women: some findings of a large national survey discussed. *Sex Marital Ther.* **10**: 169–188.

Wright AL (1983) A cross-cultural comparison of menopausal symptoms. *Med. Anthropol.* **7**: 20–35.

6

Principles of Hormone Replacement Therapy

Women approaching their fifties today are facing decisions that were not considered by a previous generation: whether or not to take hormone replacement therapy (HRT); whether to take it for relief of menopausal symptoms, or for the longer-term benefits to the skeletal and cardiovascular systems.

The media and, in particular, women's magazines frequently publish articles about the menopause and HRT. Unfortunately they are not always balanced or accurate and women are often left feeling even more confused about the subject. The decision to take HRT is not always a simple one and some women find it difficult to obtain the information they need to make an informed choice.

Health professionals, too, are not always up to date. HRT is a rapidly changing field: more and more products are reaching the marketplace and more research is being performed to establish risks and benefits so that women can be confident in the treatment they are offered. This chapter is intended to given an overview of HRT – what it is, risks and benefits, contraindications and side-effects – and to review the various methods of giving HRT.

WHAT IS HRT?

HRT usually consists of the two hormones, oestrogen and progestogen. It is the oestrogen that reportedly confers benefits to many body systems and that effectively relieves acute menopausal symptoms. Women who have had a hysterectomy can safely take oestrogen on its own, but women with a uterus are generally prescribed both hormones, as oestrogen alone has been demonstrated to increase the likelihood of endometrial hyperplasia (Henderson, 1989). Adding a progestogen, either cyclically or continuously, has been shown to protect the endometrium from hyperplastic changes (Whitehead et al 1990). This was confirmed by the Postmenopausal Estrogen/Progestin Intervention (PEPI) trial (Writing Group 1996).

Oestrogens used in HRT are **natural** rather than **synthetic** (Table 6.1). 17β-Estradiol, estrone and estriol are all types of natural oestrogen used in HRT. When given as HRT, levels of oestrogen in the blood rise to levels similar to a premenopausal level. HRT also prevents the fluctuations of oestrogen levels that are common around the time of the menopause and that often given rise to

Table 6.1 Types of oestrogen	
Natural	**Synthetic**
17β-Estradiol	Ethinylestradiol
Estradiol valerate	Mestranol
Estrone piperazine sulfate	Diethylstilbestrol

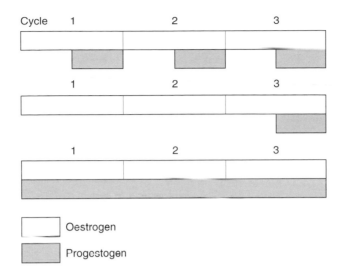

Figure 6.1 Regimens of oestrogen and progestogen in HRT.

acute menopausal symptoms. Synthetic oestrogens such as those used in the contraceptive pill (e.g. ethinylestradiol) are not used in modern forms of HRT because of the increased risk of thrombosis and hypertension (Upton 1988). Conjugated oestrogens are used in some forms of HRT. These act in a similar way to natural oestrogens and are therefore classified as natural (Stern 1982).

In clinical practice there is little difference between the natural oestrogens, all of which appear to be equally effective (Mashchak et al 1982). No one form of natural oestrogen is better than another, although individual women may prefer one to another. The aim of HRT is to provide a level of circulating oestrogen that is sufficient to relieve symptoms and also to protect against cardiovascular disease and osteoporosis. For most women this is achieved by standard doses of HRT.

HRT REGIMENS

Oestrogen therapy can be given cyclically or continuously. It is most common for oestrogen to be given on a continuous basis in order to maintain blood levels and to prevent symptoms returning. In the UK, most preparations provide continuous oestrogen therapy. Progestogen can be given cyclically, continuously or tricyclically (Fig. 6.1).

ROUTES OF ADMINISTRATION

HRT can be given in various ways (Fig. 6.2, Table 6.2). There is no ideal way of giving HRT and, for many women, the final choice should be an individual one, made in consultation with the supervising doctor. Occasionally there will be medical reasons for choosing one method over another, but in many instances the decision

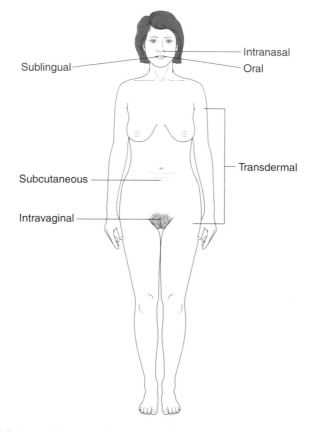

Figure 6.2 Potential routes of oestrogen administration.

Table 6.2 Routes of HRT administration	
Oestrogen	**Progestogen**
Tablet	Tablet
Patch	Patch
Gel	(Intrauterine system – not licensed for HRT)
Implant	Vaginal progesterone gel
Intranasal	
Vaginal treatments	

should reflect the treatment that the individual woman is likely to use and that is therefore most likely to be effective.

Whichever method of giving oestrogen is chosen (except local vaginal treatment), the effect on the uterus is the same, so women with a uterus should be given progestogen as well.

The first-pass effect

The main difference between oral and non-oral routes of HRT is the avoidance of the 'first pass' effects on the liver with non-oral routes. Estradiol given by tablet will pass through both the gut and the liver, resulting in a substantial part being converted into a less potent hormone (Lievertz 1987). There is wide variation in the rate of absorption between individuals and so the dose requirement for individual women will vary.

Theoretically, the first-pass effect could produce unwanted changes in the liver; whether such changes are clinically relevant to most women is unclear (Whitehead & Godfree 1992).

Tablets

Tablets are a common way of taking HRT and have been available longer than any other method. They are available in varying doses and in combination with a variety of progestogens. Some are conveniently packaged for easy compliance, whereas others can be tailored to an individual's requirements (Fig. 6.3).

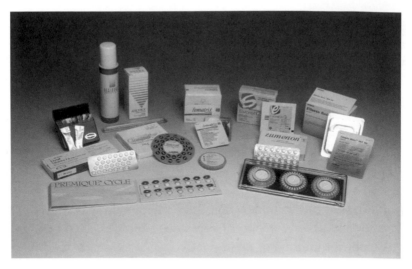

Figure 6.3 There is a wide variety of HRT available. Courtesy of the Medical Illustration Department, Northwick Park Hospital, Harrow.

Patches

Patches containing estradiol deliver a constant dose over 24 hours and are changed once or twice weekly. There are two basic types of patch: the reservoir and the matrix patch (Fig. 6.4).

Patches are worn on the buttocks or abdomen, and are generally kept in place during swimming and bathing. Reservoir patches stick

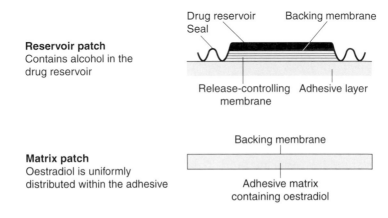

Reservoir patch
Contains alcohol in the drug reservoir

Drug reservoir   Backing membrane
Seal

Release-controlling   Adhesive layer
membrane

Matrix patch
Oestradiol is uniformly distributed within the adhesive

Backing membrane

Adhesive matrix
containing oestradiol

Figure 6.4 Reservoir and matrix patches.

less well and some women find it easier to remove the patch before swimming or bathing rather than risk losing it. Occasionally women show an allergic reaction to the patch, developing a redness and irritation under the patch, which often persists even after the patch has been removed. Matrix patches seem to cause less irritation. Women who are allergic to reservoir patches may not be allergic to matrix ones.

Most patches contain only oestrogen but there is an oestrogen–progestogen combination patch, which avoids the need for tablets at all. Patches are also available in compliance kits containing progestogen tablets for non-hysterectomized women. Patches are available in both cyclical and continuous oestrogen–progestogen regimens.

Gel

Estradiol-containing gels are available which are gently rubbed into the skin on a daily basis. The gel should preferably be applied to the upper arms or inner thighs (Fig. 6.5). It is administered in a measured dose from a pressurized canister or dosing sachet. Women should be encouraged to apply the gel over a defined area for maximum absorption. If a woman has not had a hysterectomy, progestogen tablets need to be added to the regimen, until combined gels become available.

Intranasal

Intranasal administration of drugs has been used successfully in other therapeutic areas and is now available as an estradiol-only HRT. Intranasal absorption is facilitated by the highly vascularized nature of the nasal mucosa. The pharmokinetics of intranasally administered estradiol differ from those of estradiol taken orally. With intranasal administration there is a rapid uptake of estradiol, with maximum plasma levels being achieved within 10–30 minutes. Within 12 hours the level has dropped back to untreated levels, but sustained relief of symptoms appears to occur with repeated doses (Studd et al 1999). As well as avoiding the first-pass

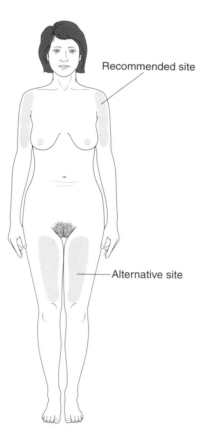

Recommended site

Alternative site

Figure 6.5 Gel should be applied widely and thinly.

effect on metabolism, nasal administration offers the benefits of simple dose adjustments, consistency of absorption and relatively easy patient administration (Studd et al 1999). A combined oestrogen–progestogen nasal spray is under investigation.

Implants

Estradiol implants are small pellets that are inserted under the skin of the buttock or abdomen, through a small incision (Fig. 6.6). The oestrogen is then released slowly over a period of months. Generally, the higher the implant dose, the longer it will remain

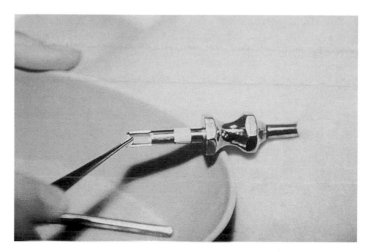

Figure 6.6 Oestrogen or testosterone implantation.

effective. Levels of oestrogen in the blood are often higher than with other routes. The hormone testosterone can also be administered by implant, either at the same time as an oestrogen implant or on its own.

There is a wide variation among women as to how long an implant will remain effective. Occasionally the physiological effect of an implant may last up to 2 years, so it is important to continue the progestogen therapy in non-hysterectomized women (Whitehead et al 1993). Rarely, a condition called **tachyphylaxis** may occur, where the woman returns for implants at increasingly shorter intervals (Ganger et al 1989). Such women experience symptoms even though their estradiol levels are raised. Repeated implants cause the levels to rise even further. So far, it is unclear whether this is harmful, but some specialists would advise caution and withhold implants if estradiol levels were very high.

Vaginal treatments

For local use, oestrogen can be administered directly to the vagina by creams, pessaries, tablets and slow-releasing rings. They exert a direct beneficial effect on atrophic vaginitis without systemic effects. These preparations are particularly useful in older women who need relief of vaginal symptoms but who are reluctant to try systemic HRT.

The oestrogens used in modern vaginal preparations are estriol and estradiol. When given at the low recommended doses for atrophic vaginitis, they are not sufficiently absorbed systemically to cause endometrial proliferation (Schmidt et al 1994). Prolonged use may lead to an endometrial effect. Vaginal oestrogens should not be used as a lubricant during sexual intercourse because of the small risk of absorption by a male partner.

Also available is a soft ring, which contains oestradiol for systemic absorption. Changed every 3 months by the woman herself, a regular dose of oestrogen is absorbed through the vagina, giving systemic relief of menopausal symptoms. When used in non-hysterectomized women, a progestogen is necessary.

Intrauterine systems

A progestogen-containing intrauterine system is available for contraceptive purposes. Research is underway looking at its use as an adjunct to oestrogen therapy as a form of hormone replacement. Such a combination may provide endometrial protection without systemic side-effects and, for many women, no bleed.

PROGESTOGENS

Progestogens are added to the treatment regimen of non-hysterectomized women to prevent endometrial hyperplasia (Grady et al 1995). Of women taking oestrogen-only therapy, 7–15% will develop endometrial hyperplasia (Sturdee et al 1978), causing irregular bleeding and the potential to progress to endometrial carcinoma (Kurman et al 1985). Adding a progestogen reduces the incidence of irregular bleeding and the risk of endometrial cancer to below those seen in untreated women (Whitehead et al 1990). Progestogens commonly used in HRT regimens are:

◆ norethisterone } testosterone derived
◆ levonorgestrel

◆ dydrogesterone } progesterone derived
◆ medroxyprogesterone acetate

If a women experiences side-effects with a progestogen, it is often worth trying one from the other group, which may not have the same effect.

Natural progesterone can be administered as a vaginal gel for use in opposition to oestrogen therapy (Casanas-Roux et al 1996). The preparation is used on alternate days for 14 days in each cycle in order to prevent endometrial proliferation. It has minimal side-effects and offers a good alternative for women who accept the vaginal route. This preparation should not be confused with natural progesterone creams used as an alternative treatment to HRT (see Ch. 8).

Cyclical progestogens

Progestogens are usually given for 10–14 days in a cycle in order to prevent endometrial stimulation. The duration of progestogen administration seems to be as important as the dose. Although it is common for progestogens to be prescribed cyclically (i.e. every 28 days), it is sometimes more convenient for a woman to take her progestogen on a calendar-month basis (i.e. a 30/31-day 'cycle'). In this instance she would take the progestogen for the first 10–14 days of each calendar month. This is much easier to remember than having to count a 28-day cycle. Cyclical progestogen results in a monthly bleed in 80–90% of women.

Doses of progestogen used in cyclical HRT are:

◆ norethisterone   1–2.5 mg
◆ dydrogesterone   10–20 mg
◆ medroxyprogesterone acetate   5–10 mg
◆ levonorgestrel   150 μg

Continuous progestogen

A continuous low dose of progestogen alongside continuous oestrogen will prevent hyperplastic changes to the endometrium without the need for a regular bleed (Archer et al 1994, Magos et al 1985). This form of therapy is suitable only for truly postmenopausal women (i.e. at least 1 year after the last menstrual bleed) because of the unacceptably high risk of irregular bleeding in perimenopausal women. In any case, irregular bleeding is common in the first few months of therapy and women should be advised of this. If they are able to persevere with the treatment, they have a good chance of experiencing amenorrhoea eventually. Continuous oestrogen–progestogen regimens are available in both tablet and patch form, or can be tailor-made with a combination of regimens.

Tricyclical progestogens (long-cycle HRT)

HRT is also administered in a regimen in which progestogen is given only every 3 months, whilst still maintaining endometrial protection (Ettinger et al 1994). This results in a bleed once every 3 months, which is apparently no heavier than a normal period (Hirvonen et al 1995). The advantage of this treatment (apart from fewer bleeds) is that potential side-effects of the progestogen are also minimized. For women who seem unable to tolerate progestogen, this is a real advantage.

Progestogen-only therapy

Women who cannot take HRT, or who prefer not to, are sometimes prescribed progestogen alone to try to alleviate vasomotor symptoms. It is not as effective as oestrogen therapy but may certainly be helpful for some women. Doses of progestogen may need to be higher than those usually given for endometrial protection (Paterson 1992, Schmidt et al 1984).

Tibolone

Tibolone is a synthetic type of HRT with oestrogenic, progestogenic and androgenic properties. It is given continuously and does not usually cause bleeding (Rymer 1992). It is effective at reducing flushes and sweats, and improves mood and libido (Benedek-Jaszmann 1987). It also protects against postmenopausal bone loss (Lyritis et al 1995). Irregular bleeding may occur in perimenopausal women (Rymer et al 1994). Episodes of bleeding in women who are more than 1 year postmenopausal should be clinically investigated.

By contrast with oestrogens, tibolone does not appear to stimulate breast tissue in the same way, although there are no data yet on the use of tibolone in women with breast cancer (Kloosterboer et al 1994). Tibolone is useful for the older women, because it may cause less breast tenderness and bleeding, which are common problems with use of HRT in older women.

SIDE-EFFECTS OF HRT

Side-effects are common in the first few weeks of starting HRT (Box 6.1). Oestrogen-related side-effects such as breast tenderness, nausea and leg cramps usually subside after 6–8 weeks on therapy. If they do not, a change in dose or type of oestrogen may be necessary.

Progestogen-related side-effects seem to be more common in cyclical regimens and often appear to be similar in type to premenstrual symptoms (e.g. irritability, anxiety, bloatedness and breast pain). They can be minimized by adjusting the dose or type of progestogen whilst ensuring that the minimum dose recommended for endometrial safety is maintained (Siddle 1989). For more information about management of side-effects, see Chapter 7.

BLEEDING PATTERNS AND HRT

Cyclical HRT

Approximately 80–90% of women who use a cyclical form of HRT experience a monthly bleed. This bleed should be regular, usually lasting between 2 and 6 days, and should not be unacceptably heavy. Mild period-type pains are common. The first few months

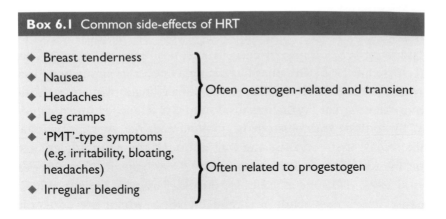

Box 6.1 Common side-effects of HRT

- Breast tenderness
- Nausea
- Headaches
- Leg cramps

⎫ Often oestrogen-related and transient

- 'PMT'-type symptoms (e.g. irritability, bloating, headaches)
- Irregular bleeding

⎫ Often related to progestogen

on treatment may not produce a regular bleed but after about three cycles the bleed should settle into a regular and predictable pattern.

Monitoring of the withdrawal bleed should take place at follow-up visits to ensure that the pattern is as expected for the regimen being prescribed (see Ch. 7 for monitoring of HRT).

Breakthrough bleeding

Breakthrough bleeding (i.e. bleeding unrelated to the progestogen course) should not occur with cyclical forms of HRT. Repeated episodes of breakthrough bleeding need to be investigated. Occasional 'one off' episodes may occur due to the following factors:

- poor compliance (particularly with the progestogen)
- drug interactions (e.g. antibiotics)
- gastrointestinal upset, leading to poor absorption of the HRT
- stress occasionally provokes bleeding, although this may be due to unintentionally missing tablets.

See Chapter 7 for management of breakthrough bleeding during use of HRT.

Continuous combined oestrogen and progestogen regimens

The aim of a continuous combined oestrogen–progestogen regimen is to avoid the need for a monthly bleed whilst maintaining endometrial safety. Some women find the thought of returning to monthly bleeds unpleasant, so the idea of a 'period-free' HRT is attractive. This is particularly true for older women starting HRT for the first time, many years after their periods have stopped. Irregular bleeding is common initially, although the incidence does decrease with length of use (Staland 1981). Women changing from a cyclical to a continuous regimen are advised to make the change at the end of a withdrawal bleed. Bleeding that occurs during the initial few months of treatment does not need investigating, but prolonged or unacceptable bleeding may require a change of treatment. If bleeding is persistent, clinical investigation will be necessary (Leather et al 1991).

CONTRAINDICATIONS TO HRT

Much confusion surrounds the issue of true contraindications to HRT. In the past, both medical professionals and the lay public have wrongly applied data relating to the oral contraceptive pill to HRT. This has led to confusion over who can and who cannot take HRT safely. Contraindications can be divided into conditions that usually lead to a woman being advised not to take HRT and those that warrant further tests or investigations before HRT is prescribed. Contraindications to HRT are (Rymer 2000):

- endometrial carcinoma
- active venous thrombosis
- severe active liver disease
- pregnancy
- otosclerosis.

History of endometrial carcinoma

Early-stage endometrial carcinoma, treated by surgical resection is not a contraindication to the use of HRT. If there was an incomplete resection or evidence of recurrence, this would be an absolute contraindication. The risk of using HRT would have to be weighed against the quality of life without it (Rymer 2000).

Active venous thrombosis

Previously, HRT was not thought to be associated with venous thrombosis. This was thought to be because HRT was a more physiological replacement of oestrogen rather than a pharmacological dose of synthetic oestrogen. Then, in 1996, three papers were published suggesting that HRT carries a threefold increase in risk (Daly et al 1996, Grodstein et al 1996, Jick et al 1996). A further study supported these findings, but suggested that most of the risk is concentrated in the first year of use (Gutthann et al 1997). For this reason, active venous thrombosis is a contraindication to the use of HRT (Rymer 2000). See also Relative contraindications below.

Liver disease

Severe, active liver disease is a contraindication to HRT (Rymer 2000). If a woman has previously had mild liver disease, it may be suggested that she has a non-oral type of HRT in order to avoid the first-pass effect on the liver.

Pregnancy

Pregnancy can occur during the perimenopausal era and, if the woman mistakes the resulting amenorrhoea as her menopause, HRT may be started inadvertently. If pregnancy is suspected, HRT should not be commenced.

Otosclerosis

This is a condition of progressive deafness that has been known to worsen during pregnancy. As no data are available regarding this condition and the use of HRT, caution is usually advised, although there is no substantial evidence to suggest a deterioration with use of HRT.

Relative contraindications

Conditions that may be considered relative contraindications are discussed below. Women with any of these conditions will sometimes be given HRT, but supervision may need to be more regular and the decision to prescribe HRT may not be straightforward. Referral to a specialist centre may be necessary and pretreatment investigations may be required. Relative contraindications are:

◆ abnormal vaginal bleeding
◆ previous localized breast cancer
◆ previous venous thrombosis
◆ fibroids
◆ endometriosis
◆ untreated hypertension.

Undiagnosed abnormal vaginal bleeding

If a woman has experienced postmenopausal bleeding (i.e. bleeding more than 12 months after her last normal period), or if she has unexplained intermenstrual or postcoital bleeding, these should be investigated before HRT is commenced. In most instances investigation will not reveal any abnormal pathology and HRT can be started.

Previous breast cancer

A recent history of breast cancer is generally considered to be a contraindication to taking HRT. With earlier detection of disease and improved therapy, breast cancer is being detected at an earlier, curable, stage. More women are therefore entering the menopause following successful treatment for breast cancer. Whether HRT is safe for these women has yet to be determined by prospective randomized studies. Retrospective analyses appear to indicate that the incidence of breast cancer recurrence in HRT users is not markedly different to that expected, regardless of hormone use. Some specialist menopause clinics would prescribe HRT to women with previous localized breast cancer, but the potential risks must be weighed against potential benefits, and the woman herself will play a crucial role in the treatment decision (Nand et al 1998).

Previous venous thrombosis

A history of venous thrombosis is the single biggest risk factor for future thrombosis, so this risk needs to be balanced against potential benefits of HRT. A positive thrombophilia screen will help to identify those women who should probably not use HRT, but a negative thrombophilia screen cannot offer complete reassurance, as women with a personal history of venous thrombosis are at risk of recurrence even if a thrombophilia screen is negative (Keeling 1999).

The Royal College of Obstetricians and Gynaecologists (1999) has issued recommendations regarding HRT and venous thrombosis as follows:

◆ There is no indication for routine screening for thrombophilia in women starting HRT.
◆ Women starting HRT should have a personal and family history taken of thromboembolic events.
◆ Women starting on HRT should have an assessment made of additional risk factors for thrombolic disease.
◆ Women with a personal or family history of venous thrombosis should undergo a thrombophilia screen.

Fibroids

After the menopause, fibroids usually shrink. The use of HRT may cause them to enlarge, causing bleeding problems and discomfort. Ultrasonographic investigation will be helpful for monitoring fibroids whilst a woman is taking HRT. Small fibroids are not generally a problem.

Endometriosis

Endometriosis is a hormone-dependent disease. Even if it has previously been treated by surgery, there is a small chance that HRT could cause it to recur. Careful monitoring is essential and women should be warned of the theoretical risk of the condition returning. Continuous combined HRT or tibolone may be recommended (Rymer 2000).

Untreated hypertension

Although HRT does not adversely affect blood pressure, it is generally advised that high blood pressure should be under control before HRT is commenced.

Other medical conditions

Gallstones

If there are pre-existing gallstones then non-oral HRT would be preferable, and in women who are not known to have gallstones oral therapy may unmask previously unknown stones (Rymer 2000).

Epilepsy

Some antiepileptic drugs will enhance the metabolism of oral oestrogen. Higher doses or non-oral oestrogen may be necessary.

Previous myocardial infarction or angina

This is controversial. HRT should be avoided during acute episodes when the patient is immobilized in bed. Most observational studies have suggested a significant effect for secondary prevention, but the Heart and Estrogen/Progestin Replacement Study (HERS), a prospective randomized study, did not confirm this (Hulley et al 1998). Further studies are underway.

Varicose veins

These are not worsened by HRT. Leg cramps are associated with HRT use, particularly in the early stages of treatment. Women themselves often perceive these as a problem and can often be reassured, provided there is no evidence of thrombosis. Varicose veins are associated with a doubling in risk of postoperative thrombosis, so the use of HRT in women undergoing surgery should be considered a risk of thrombosis and precautionary measures taken.

Heavy smokers

Women should be encouraged to stop smoking for general health reasons, but a heavy smoker can still take HRT. Cardiovascular benefits would be even greater if the woman could also give up smoking. If a woman is experiencing profound menopausal symptoms, it may not be a diplomatic time to suggest that she should stop smoking!

Migraine

It is impossible to predict the effect of HRT on migraine. A trial of therapy may be necessary. Some women find that migraines improve after the menopause.

Diabetes

Diabetic women can safely take HRT, but glucose levels should be monitored in the early months of treatment in case adjustment of insulin is required. Theoretically, non-oral routes may be preferable.

THE BREAST ISSUE

Breast cancer is a common disease and appears to be hormone related. Known risk factors for breast cancer are:

◆ early menarche
◆ late first pregnancy
◆ late menopause
◆ obesity (associated with higher levels of circulating oestrogen).

Anxiety about breast cancer and HRT is legitimate. Little agreement has been reached through clinical trials, although a large number of studies have been performed. Some studies have shown a slight increase in risk with HRT use (Colditz et al 1990, Harris et al 1992), whereas others have seen no change (Dupont & Page 1991, Yang et al 1992). The addition of a progestogen to oestrogen does not reduce the risk of breast cancer among postmenopausal women (Colditz et al 1995). In 1997, the Collaborative Group on Hormonal Factors in Breast Cancer published data on analysis of 52 705 women with and 108 411 women without breast cancer, from 51 studies in 21 countries. The outcomes of this analysis showed that the risk of breast cancer increases slightly in women using HRT and that the risk increases the longer treatment is used (Collaborative Group 1997). The risk of breast cancer in non-users of HRT is calculated as 45 cases per 1000 women aged 50–70 years. Extrapolating from the findings of the above analysis, the use of HRT for 5 years would be expected to result in the diagnosis of 2 extra breast cancer cases by the age of 70 years. Use of HRT for 10 years would mean an extra 6 cases per 1000 women, and for 15 years an extra 12 cases (Collaborative Group 1997).

If a woman develops breast cancer while taking HRT, the prognosis may be better than if she had not been taking the HRT (Bergkfist et al 1989). Whether this is a true effect of HRT, or whether it is due to the increased surveillance of women on HRT, is unclear. Neither is it of much consolation to a woman herself if she should develop a malignancy.

Family history of breast cancer

A woman with a strong family history of breast cancer is already at an increased risk herself. There is no evidence that such women increase their risk further if they take HRT, but few studies have been carried out. These women are often prescribed HRT after a full and frank discussion of the possible risks and with particular attention being paid to breast surveillance. If a woman has two or more first-degree relatives with breast cancer under the age of 45 years, then she could be referred for genetic counselling to test for *BRCA1* and *BRCA2* genes. This may make her decision about HRT easier. For further information about breast monitoring, see Chapter 7.

DURATION OF TREATMENT

How long a woman chooses to stay on HRT will depend largely on her reasons for taking it. Women with acute symptoms may need HRT for only a year or so before symptoms resolve. Others may stop HRT after 2 years, only to find that menopausal symptoms return because they are still in the climacteric phase.

For long-term protection of heart and bone, treatment is recommended for at least 5 years. Women wanting to stay on HRT for more than 10 years need an open discussion with regard to risks and benefits, particularly in relation to breast cancer. Currently, many women take HRT for only a few months because of unacceptable side-effects. Although this is a personal decision, women should be encouraged to return for a consultation before stopping HRT. A change in regimen may be all that is needed to enable her to continue with confidence.

How to stop

Women wanting to stop HRT may fear that their symptoms will suddenly return. If HRT is stopped suddenly, some women experience symptoms as a result of the rapidly falling oestrogen levels. This will depend on the dose of oestrogen she has been using and for how long she has been using it. For this reason it is often suggested that the oestrogen be tailed off gradually over a period of a few weeks. Initially the dose can be reduced, then tablets can be taken on alternate days or patches changed less frequently. Meanwhile the progestogen is continued as normal. Once all oestrogen has been stopped, the progestogen can be discontinued at the end of a course. Women discontinuing HRT after having oestrogen implants should be advised to continue progestogen until withdrawal bleeding ceases.

REFERENCES

Archer DF, Pickar JH, Bottiglioni F et al (1994) Bleeding patterns in post-menopausal women taking continuous combined or sequential regimens of conjugated estrogens with medoxyprogesterone acetate. *Obstet. Gynecol.* **83**: 686–692.

Benedek-Jaszmann LJ (1987) Long term placebo controlled efficacy and safety study of ORG OD 14 in climacteric women. *Maturitas* Suppl 1: 25–33.

Bergkfist L, Adami HO, Persson I et al (1989) The risk of breast cancer in post-menopausal women who have used estrogen replacement therapy. *J. Am. Med. Assoc.* **321**: 293–297.

Casanas-Roux F, Nisolle M, Marbaix E et al (1996) Morphometric, immunohisto-logical and three-dimensional evaluation of the endometrium of menopausal women treated by oestrogen and Crinone, a new slow release vaginal proges-terone. *Hum. Reprod.* **11**: 357–363.

Colditz GA, Stampfer MJ, Wilett WC et al (1990) Prospective study of estrogen replacement therapy and risk of breast cancer in postmenopausal women. *J. Am. Med. Assoc.* **264**: 2648–2653.

Colditz GA, Hankinson SE, Hunter DJ et al (1995) The use of oestrogen and progestins and the risk of breast cancer in postmenopausal women. *N. Engl. J. Med.* **332**: 1589–1593.

Collaborative Group on Hormonal Factors in Breast Cancer (1997) Breast cancer and HRT: collaborative reanalysis of data from 51 epidemiological studies of 52 705 women with breast cancer and 108 411 women without breast cancer. *Lancet* **350**: 1047–1059.

Daly E, Vessey MP, Hawkins MM et al (1996) Risk of venous thromboembolism in users of hormone replacement therapy. *Lancet* **348**: 977–980.

Dupont WD, Page DL (1991) Menopausal estrogen replacement therapy and breast cancer. *Arch. Intern. Med.* **151**: 67–72.

Ettinger B, Selby J, Citron JT (1994) Cyclic HRT using quarterly progestin. *Obstet. Gynecol.* **83**: 693–700.

Gangar K, Cust M, Whitehead MI (1989) Symptoms of oestrogen deficiency with supraphysiological levels of plasma oestradiol concentrations in women with oestradiol implants. *Br. Med. J.* **299**: 601.

Grady D, Gebretsadik T, Kerilowske K et al (1995) HRT and endometrial cancer risk: a meta analysis. *Obstet. Gynecol.* **85**: 304–313.

Grodstein F, Stampfer MJ, Goldhaber SZ et al (1996) Prospective study of exoge-nous hormones and risk of pulmonary embolism. *Lancet* **348**: 983–987.

Gutthann SP, Rodriquez LAG, Castellsagne J, Oliart AD (1997) HRT and the risk of venous thromboembolism: population based case control study. *Br. Med. J.* **314**: 796–800.

Harris RE, Namboodiri KK, Wynder EL (1992) Breast cancer risk: effects of estro-gen replacement therapy and body mass. *J. Natl. Cancer Inst.* **84**: 1575–1582.

Henderson BE (1989) The cancer question: an overview of recent epidemiologi-cal and retrospective data. *Am. J. Obstet. Gynecol.* **161**: 1859.

Hirvonen E, Salmi T, Puolakka J et al (1995) Can progestin be limited to every third month only in postmenopausal women taking estrogen? *Maturitas* **21**: 39–44.

Hulley S, Grady D, Bush T et al (1998) Randomised trial of estrogen and progestogen for secondary prevention of coronary heart disease in postmenopausal women. *J. Am. Med. Assoc.* **280**: 605–613.

Jick H, Derby L, Myers MW et al (1996) Risk of hospital admission for ideopathic venous thromboembolism among users of postmenopausal oestrogens. *Lancet* **348**: 981–983.

Keeling D (1999) HRT and venous thromboembolism. *Br. J. Menopause Soc.* **5**(3): 135–136.

Kloosterboer HJ, Schoonen WGEJ, Deckers GH, Kiljn JGM (1994) Effects of progestogens and ORG OD14 on in vitro and in vivo tumour models. *J. Steroid Biochem. Mol. Biol.* **49**: 311–318.

Kurman RJ, Kaminski PF, Norris RJ (1985) The behavior of endometrial hyperplasia – a long term study of untreated hyperplasia in 170 patients. *Cancer* **56**: 403–412.

Leather AT, Savvas M, Studd JWW (1991) Endometrial histology and bleeding patterns after 8 years of continuous combined estrogen and progestogen therapy in postmenopausal women. *Obstet. Gynecol.* **6**: 1008–1010.

Lievertz RW (1987) Pharmacology and pharmokinetics of oestrogens. *Am. J. Obstet. Gynecol.* **156**: 1289–1293.

Lyritis GP, Karpathios S, Basdekis K et al (1995) Prevention of post-oophorectomy bone loss with tibolone. *Maturitas* **22**: 247–253.

Magos AL, Brincat M, Studd JWW et al (1985) Amenorrhoea and endometrial atrophy with continuous oral oestrogen and progestogen therapy in postmenopausal women. *Obstet. Gynecol.* **65**: 496–499.

Mashchak CA, Lobo RA, Dozono-Takano R et al (1982) Comparison of pharmacodynamic properties of various oestrogen formulations. *Am. J. Obstet. Gynecol.* **144**: 511–518.

Nand SL, Eden JA, Wren BG (1998) Estrogens after breast cancer. In: Studd JW (ed.) *The Management of the Menopause, Annual Review*, pp. 199–210. Parthenon, London.

Paterson MEL (1992) A randomised double blind cross over trial into the effects of norethisterone on climacteric symptoms and biochemical profiles. *Br. J. Obstet. Gynaecol.* **89**: 464–472.

Royal College of Obstetricians and Gynaecologists (1999) *Hormone Replacement Therapy and Venous Thromboembolism Guidelines*, No. 19. RCOG, London.

Rymer J (1992) Tibolone: alternative relief for postmenopausal symptoms. *J. Sex. Health* **2**(5): 25–27.

Rymer J (2000) Relative and absolute contraindications to HRT. In: Studd JWW (ed.) *The Management of the Menopause, Millenium Review*, pp. 21–26. Parthenon, London.

Rymer J, Fogelman I, Chapman MG (1994) The incidence of vaginal bleeding with tibolone treatment. *Br. J. Obstet. Gynaecol.* **101**: 53–56.

Schmidt G, Andersson SB, Nordle O et al (1994) Release of 17beta oestradiol from a vaginal ring in postmenopausal women: a pharmokinetic evaluation. *Gynecol. Obstet. Invest.* **38**: 253–260.

Siddle NC (1989) Psychological effects of different progestogens. Consensus Development Conference on Progestogens. *International Proceedings Journal* **1**: 214–217.

Staland B (1981) Continuous treatment with natural oestrogen and progestogens. A method to avoid endometrial stimulation. *Maturitas* **3**: 145.

Stern MD (1982) Pharmacology of conjugated oestrogens. *Maturitas* **4**: 333–339.

Studd J, Pornel B, Marton I et al (1999) Efficacy and acceptability of intranasal 17beta oestradiol for menopausal symptoms: randomised dose–response study. *Lancet* **353**: 1574–1578.

Sturdee DW, Wade-Evans T, Paterson MEL et al (1978) Relations between bleeding pattern, endometrial histology and oestrogen treatment in postmenopausal women. *Br. Med. J.* i: 1575–1577.

Upton V (1988) Contraception in the woman over 40. In: Studd JWW, Whitehead MI (eds) *The Menopause*, pp. 289–304. Blackwell Scientific, Oxford.

Whitehead MI, Godfree V (1992) *Hormone Replacement Therapy – Your Questions Answered*. Churchill Livingstone, London.

Whitehead MI, Hillard TC, Crook D (1990) The role and use of progestogens. *Obstet. Gynecol.* **75** (Suppl 4): 59–71s.

Whitehead MI, Whitcroft SJ, Hillard TC (1993) *Atlas of the Menopause*. Encyclopaedia of Visual Medicine Series no. 25. Parthenon, London.

Writing Group of the PEPI Trial (1996) Effects of hormone replacement therapy on endometrial histology in postmenopausal women: The Postmenopausal Estrogen/Progestin Intervention (PEPI) trial. *J. Am. Med. Assoc.* **275**: 370–375.

Yang CT, Daling JR, Band PR et al (1992) Non contraceptive hormone use and risk of breast cancer. *Cancer, Causes Control* **3**: 475–479.

7

Practical Aspects of Hormone Replacement Therapy

Ten years ago, the prescription of hormone replacement therapy (HRT) and discussion of menopause issues was confined mainly to brief consultations with general practitioners or occasional visits to gynaecology departments. Women experiencing severe menopausal symptoms might have received HRT, but other women simply 'put up with the symptoms'. If a woman sought the help of her doctor, she was fortunate if she got more than a 5-minute consultation and a prescription.

Fortunately, times have changed in all areas of medicine and perhaps women's health is one area that has seen more changes than any other. Women themselves are demanding an improved service from healthcare professionals, particularly when it comes to issues such as the menopause. The choice of whether to take HRT has, to a large extent, been removed from the prescriber to the individual woman, who now makes the choice herself after consideration of all the necessary information and facts. The doctor still has the final say after assessing the woman, but the decision is more likely to have been made jointly, after greater discussion between doctor and patient.

The nurse, particularly the practice nurse, sits conveniently between patient and doctor. She is often the facilitator in the decision-making process. The woman will not take HRT until she has all the information she needs and the doctor will not prescribe it unless confident that it is safe and appropriate. The nurse can be involved both in helping the woman to make an informed choice and in ensuring that the necessary procedures are carried out before treatment starts. In future, nurses themselves could be the prescribers as nurse prescribing becomes available. Broadly speaking the nurse's role falls into three categories:

◆ informing women about the menopause and its effects, and discussing therapy options
◆ preparing a woman to take HRT or other therapies
◆ monitoring and assessing the woman taking treatment.

INFORMING WOMEN

Before a woman can make what is described as an 'informed choice', she needs the necessary information to help her make the decision wisely (Fig. 7.1). Many women discover that gathering accurate information about the menopause and treatment options is a difficult task. They often have to choose between a medical textbook, which is dauntingly detailed, or a magazine article that emphasizes either the horrors or the miracles of HRT. Balanced articles and books are hard to find if you are not sure where to start looking.

Increasingly, the nurse in general practice is becoming the person to whom women will turn for unbiased but accurate knowledge. It is therefore vital that nurses are well informed about the availability of treatments, the risks and benefits of HRT, and that

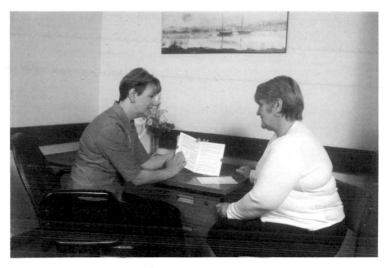

Figure 7.1 Informing women helps them to make an informed decision. Courtesy of the Medical Illustration Department, Northwick Park Hospital, Harrow.

they keep up to date with current research. The subject of menopause is a vast one, so what do you choose to tell women and how do you impart the information? How do you ensure that the women who really need the information receive it, and how do you reach across barriers of class, education and race so that all women have the necessary information for themselves?

Issues to cover when considering what women need to know in order to make an informed choice about therapy options include:

◆ understanding the menopause and its effects
◆ dispelling myths about the menopause and treatments
◆ unrealistic expectations, particularly of HRT
◆ understanding HRT and other therapies
◆ anticipating anxieties
◆ promoting health and well-being beyond the menopause.

Understanding the menopause

It is sometimes necessary to spend time explaining about the female reproductive system so that each woman has a better understanding about what is happening to her body. Women may need information about changes that occur and symptoms they may experience. For some women this will enable them to have a better understanding of HRT and how it is used. Discussions about fluctuating hormone levels and changing period patterns may be helpful to some, whilst other women may want more in-depth discussion about osteoporosis or risk of cardiovascular disease after menopause.

Dispelling myths

There are many old wives' tales about the menopause and many beliefs about HRT that are widely held but inaccurate. These need to be discussed and corrected. Some of the myths relate to a misunderstanding about what HRT actually does, while the old wives' tales may be passed from mother to daughter or from friend to friend. Repeated often enough they begin to sound like authoritative statements and can be difficult to dispel.

If you started your periods late, you will get a bad (or good) menopause.
Age of menarche has no influence on subsequent menopausal symptoms.

If your mother had a bad menopause, then you will too.
This is not necessarily true, although a particularly early or late menopause may run in families.

If you live a healthy lifestyle, you can avoid unpleasant menopausal symptoms.
If only this were true! Menopausal symptoms may affect the fittest and healthiest women as well as the 'couch potatoes'. A healthy lifestyle is always to be commended but will not guarantee you a trouble-free menopause.

If you could not take the contraceptive pill, then you cannot take HRT. This is a widely held belief that has arisen from a basic misunderstanding about how HRT differs from the contraceptive pill.

If you have never been pregnant you will have a delayed menopause. This is untrue; parity is unrelated to time of menopause.

If you take HRT, you will simply make things worse when you stop. HRT does not postpone symptoms, but overrides them, so provided treatment is taken for long enough, symptoms should not be worse when HRT is stopped.

These and other myths about menopause and HRT are commonplace and it can be a hard job convincing women that medical knowledge has improved and that research changed our practice over the years. This is one reason for providing good-quality literature about the subject so that women can take it away, read it and return with the questions.

Unrealistic expectations

The glamour issue

Some women start HRT with false expectations of what it will do for them. They may have read media reports of how HRT will keep them young and be hoping that the wrinkles and greying hairs will disappear. If so, they are certain to be disappointed when they discover that, even after taking HRT, they do not look 10 years younger! However, HRT may have a positive effect on sleep pattern, perhaps making the woman look and feel less tired and giving her more energy to live her life. It is helpful to have discussed this issue, particularly with women who seem to be asking for HRT primarily for this reason.

Which symptoms will be improved?

There are some symptoms that are very common at the time of the menopause and that respond very well to HRT in nearly all women, for example hot flushes and night sweats. Other symptoms can arise at this time that may or may not respond to HRT, depending on the underlying cause. An example would be poor memory: some women find that this improves with HRT, others do not, and it would be wrong to mislead women into thinking that all loss of memory will improve once HRT is started. It is well worth taking the time to help the woman consider her symptoms and try to assess which are likely to improve with HRT and which are not. No promises can be made, but after discussion it sometimes transpires that certain symptoms have not actually arisen at this time, but have always been a problem. In this case it is unlikely that HRT will help.

Hot flushes are usually the first symptoms to improve with HRT use; other symptoms may take much longer. Women should be warned that their symptoms will not disappear overnight but that some symptoms may take weeks or even months to improve:

◆ Vasomotor symptoms may take 2–3 months to improve.
◆ Urogenital symptoms may take 4–6 months.
◆ Psychological symptoms may take 6–9 months.

Understanding HRT

The word 'hormone' can be off-putting to some women as they associate it with harmful and unwanted effects. Women who are familiar with the contraceptive pill may confuse it with hormone replacement therapy and draw the wrong conclusions about HRT. The woman who is told at age 35 years to stop the contraceptive pill because she is a smoker will be confused when at the age of 50 years she is advised to consider HRT in order to promote health. A simple explanation about the difference between 'synthetic' and 'natural' HRT is required.

Most women will understand that HRT consists of oestrogen, but some may not realize that progestogen is also often given. It is important that the woman who has not had a hysterectomy understands the need for a progestogen alongside the oestrogen. Women should be warned of the possible effects of the progestogen, and in particular the likely timing of the withdrawal bleed, if appropriate. Once it has been decided which HRT a woman will take, it is helpful to explain to her which part of the treatment is oestrogen and which is progestogen. This will enable her to identify clearly the components of her own treatment and so be able to relate the side-effects to one or other component. It also means that with some therapies she will be able occasionally to alter the timing of her bleed if it is inconvenient. Most HRT preparations are packaged in a 'user friendly' way, but women may still need an explanation of how to take the treatment. This is especially so for the non-oral preparations, which are a less familiar way of taking medication for most women.

Many women do not realize that HRT is not simply one medication but a variety of doses, types and regimens. It is important to stress to women that the first preparation they try may not be the one that is most suited to them and that some adjustment or 'tailoring' of the dose may be necessary.

Concern about side-effects is one of the commonest reasons given for stopping HRT (Newton et al 1997). Yet, in many instances, it is not the actual side-effects that are unbearable (although this is occasionally the case), but rather the underlying anxieties caused by the side-effects which make a woman consider stopping her HRT. For example, the woman with breast tenderness fears that she may be getting breast cancer; the woman with leg cramps fears she is developing a thrombosis; and the woman with headaches is frightened of having a stroke.

Side-effects in the early weeks of starting any form of HRT are common and you should prepare women to experience them. They usually subside on their own, but occasionally a change in dosage or type of HRT is required. Women who are prepared for these early side-effects are more likely to stay on the treatment if they understand that they are common and not dangerous. With as many as two-thirds of women stopping HRT in the first 6 months (Hall & Spector 1992), primarily because of side-effects, it is particularly important that those who are recommended HRT for osteoporosis or cardiovascular protection realize that short-term HRT is unlikely to confer much benefit. These women, especially, should be encouraged to return to the clinic if they have problems, rather than simply stopping treatment.

Anticipating anxieties

When a woman comes to discuss the issue of HRT it is likely that she will have lots of questions to ask and perhaps some concerns to express. Some women will have anxieties in their mind that they are hesitant to raise, either because they do not want to look foolish or simply because they are hoping that you will raise it first. It is therefore helpful to address commonly held anxieties with all women, as well as encouraging women to ask specifically about issues that are of concern to them individually. Such issues are described below.

Fear of cancer

The issue of cancer, and in particular breast cancer, is very important to all women. This fear is not helped by many media articles that have exacerbated fears by printing 'scare stories' that are biased or unproven. Even if the matter is not raised by a woman herself, it is a good subject to discuss as it gives the opportunity for education about 'breast awareness' and stressing the need for mammography in women over 50 years old. It is reassuring to be able to remind women that a balanced form of HRT, containing oestrogen and progestogen, will prevent a build-up of the womb lining and so reduce risk of endometrial cancer. You can also advise her that the risk of female cancers, such as those of the ovary, cervix and fallopian tubes, is not increased with the use of HRT. For information on HRT and the risk of breast cancer, see Chapter 6.

Weight gain

Many women fear that by starting HRT they will suddenly have a dramatic uncontrollable rise in weight. For the woman already facing a struggle with her weight, the prospect of gaining more can be quite alarming. There is certainly no evidence that HRT causes a significant weight gain in most women taking it. Some women do gain weight after starting HRT, but it is impossible to know whether the HRT itself was the cause. A general discussion about nutrition, energy requirements and exercise is helpful.

Bleeding

The return of a monthly bleed is a major drawback with many types of HRT. Studies suggest that bleeding is an important reason for stopping HRT in short- and long-term users (Karakoc & Erenus 1998, Ulrich et al 1997). This has significant implications for long-term usage and therefore the long-term benefits to health. You should warn women when to expect their bleed, reassuring them that it should not be too heavy or painful and that if the regimen is carefully balanced the bleed will be easily predicted each month. If a woman is truly postmenopausal (as opposed to perimenopausal), you should discuss the option of a 'no-bleed' treatment (see Ch. 6). Higher rates of continuation have been achieved with appropriately used continuous combined preparations (Rymer 1998).

Fertility

You should remind women that HRT will not act as a contraceptive: the perimenopausal woman will need to continue using a contraceptive method whilst taking HRT (see Ch. 5). However, you can also reassure the postmenopausal woman that the return of a monthly bleed does not indicate the return of fertility.

Promoting health and well-being

For many women, the menopause and its accompanying symptoms may be the trigger for a woman to evaluate her health and make decisions about her future lifestyle. Health professionals can give information on many issues relating to good health, including smoking cessation, nutrition, exercise and stress reduction. This may be a good opportunity to discuss screening tests available such as mammography and cervical cytology. Helping women to look beyond the menopause, to an increased quality and quantity of life, because of changes made at this time is important.

INFORMATION – HOW WILL YOU GIVE IT?

Once you have decided that you want to improve awareness among all women approaching the menopause with whom you have contact, you are faced with trying to decide the best way of doing it. There is in fact no 'best' way, and you may need to experiment to see what works best for you and your clients. Many ways have been tried, and what is successful in one area of practice may not work well somewhere else. Here are a few ideas that other nurses have used; you may like to try them yourself or perhaps adapt them to your own situation.

Ideas for providing information
◆ Group sessions (open or by invitation)
◆ Individual targeting of women (by age or risk assessment)
◆ Loan of books and videos
◆ Free literature
◆ Dedicated clinic session (open or by invitation)
◆ Opportunistic moments.

These are discussed more fully in Chapter 9.

PREPARING A WOMAN TO TAKE HRT

Any woman who has made the decision to consider HRT, ideally after being fully informed, wants to be sure that the treatment will be safe for her and that she will be adequately monitored whilst on therapy. Certain tests are often carried out before HRT is prescribed and while the woman is taking it. It often falls to the nurse to carry out these tests and to answer questions arising from them.

Investigations before HRT
There are guidelines on how women on HRT should be monitored and what investigations should be done before its prescription.

Box 7.1 Investigations to consider before starting HRT

◆ Medical history
◆ Symptom history
◆ Height and weight measurement
◆ Blood pressure determination
◆ Breast examination
◆ Pelvic examination

Research indicates that this varies between different health professionals (Andersson et al 1998). The following are to be considered, as listed in Box 7.1.

Medical history

In general practice, a full medical history will already be available in the patient's records, but at other clinics it will be necessary to ask the patient directly about issues that might contraindicate the use of HRT. It may also reveal other reasons why HRT should be considered, such as a family history of heart disease or osteoporosis. After taking a full history, the nurse or doctor may decide that further investigations are required before HRT is started.

Symptom history

If a woman is presenting with climacteric symptoms, it may seem obvious to give her time to describe them. However, women themselves have complained that they often have little opportunity to talk about what they are experiencing. A 'listening ear' can be therapeutic in itself, and for some women the reassurance that what they are experiencing is common is enough to alleviate anxiety. Taking a good history before treatment also helps to evaluate the effectiveness of treatment at a later date. Symptom charts and questionnaires can be helpful in some circumstances.

Height and weight

A baseline height measurement will be useful for monitoring purposes if a woman is at high risk of osteoporosis. Measuring weight as well enables you to calculate body mass index, which is useful for general health advice. If a woman is very overweight or underweight you may decide to offer specific help with this issue, but it is unlikely to influence the prescribing of HRT. Another reason to measure a woman's weight is so that there is a record of her pretreatment weight if she thinks the HRT is causing her to gain weight.

Breast examination

We have an ethical responsibility to advise women of the increased risk of breast cancer associated with the long-term use of HRT. The prescribing doctor may perform a breast examination if clinically indicated in order to rule out any pre-existing lumps or abnormalities, which would need investigation before HRT was started. Mammography is not routinely recommended before starting HRT, except for women considered to be at a high risk for breast cancer. All women over 50 years should be encouraged to have 3-yearly mammograms as recommended by the guidelines of the National Breast Screening programme, whether or not they are taking HRT (Fig. 7.2).

Pelvic examination

Bimanual pelvic examination may be performed, if clinically indicated, before starting HRT. Clinical indications for pelvic examination include the presence of fibroids or ovarian cysts, abnormal vaginal bleeding or pelvic pain. If any abnormality is found, it should be investigated before HRT is started. Additional cervical smears are unnecessary unless clinically indicated.

Extra investigations

The following extra investigations may be required:

◆ thyroid function tests

- ◆ thrombophilia screen
- ◆ lipid profile
- ◆ mammography
- ◆ follicle stimulating hormone level
- ◆ bone densitometry
- ◆ endometrial assessment.

Thyroid function testing

Symptoms of thyroid deficiency may be similar to climacteric symptoms and often affect women in mid life, so occasionally thyroid function tests are performed to make a differential diagnosis.

Thrombophilia screen

This is important for women who have had a previous thrombosis, or who have a strong family history of thrombosis (see Ch. 6).

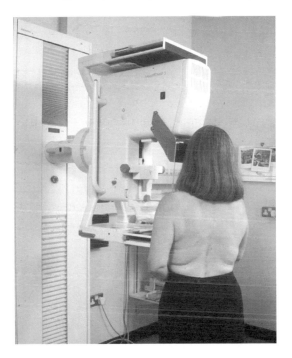

Figure 7.2 Mammography. Courtesy of the Medical Illustration Department, Northwick Park Hospital, Harrow.

Lipid profile

This is useful in women who have a strong family history of heart disease. The results may provide an indication *for* HRT rather than against it.

Mammography

All women aged over 50 years are encouraged to be part of the National Breast Screening programme. Women over 65 years can elect to continue having mammograms every 3 years, on request. They will not receive regular recalls.

The Royal College of Radiologists (1998) recommends that 'commencement of HRT is not an indication for baseline mammography. There is no evidence to suggest that mammography is cost effective in this situation and routine mammography outside of the national Breast Screening Programme is not justified'.

Under the age of 50 years, women starting HRT should be offered mammography if they have significant risk factors for breast cancer, such as a history of benign breast disease with atypia or a first-degree relative with premenopausal breast cancer (Page & Glasier 2000).

Follicle stimulating hormone level

Measurement of follicle stimulating hormone (FSH) levels is useful in the hysterectomized woman who is experiencing less typical climacteric symptoms, and is important in the diagnosis of premature menopause. A single determination of FSH level is unlikely to be reliable, so serial measurements should be performed.

Bone densitometry

If available, bone densitometry is useful for women who may be at risk of osteoporosis but who will take HRT only if that risk could be demonstrated. (See Ch. 3 for indications for bone densitometry.)

Endometrial assessment

If a woman has experienced abnormal bleeding, such as heavy prolonged periods, or if she has had a postmenopausal bleed (i.e. 12 months or more since her last period), assessment of the endometrium may be required. An endometrial sample may be taken or ultrasonography used to measure the endometrial thickness.

In most instances the primary healthcare team will carry out the relevant tests, but some women may need referral to a specialist menopause clinic. These might include:

◆ women with previous breast cancer or a first-degree relative with the disease
◆ women with a history of several episodes of thrombosis
◆ women with a complicated medical history
◆ women with a premature menopause
◆ women with concurrent gynaecological problems, such as fibroids, endometriosis or abnormal bleeding
◆ women who have already tried many types of HRT with little success.

MONITORING AND EVALUATION OF HRT

Initial evaluation should be offered to women after about 3–4 months on therapy, or after changing to a new regimen (Box 7.2). By this time, early side-effects should have subsided and a regular pattern of bleeding should be established with a cyclical regimen. If side-effects have persisted after this time, it may be necessary to consider a change of regimen.

Once a woman is established on a satisfactory treatment, with few side-effects and an acceptable bleed, if appropriate, follow-up visits can be reduced to twice a year, or sooner if problems arise.

> **Box 7.2** Ongoing assessments for women on HRT
>
> ◆ Weight
> ◆ Blood pressure
> ◆ Symptom assessment
> ◆ Side-effect assessment
> ◆ Monitoring of bleeding
> ◆ Breast examination, if appropriate
> ◆ Pelvic examination, if appropriate
> ◆ Question time

Ongoing assessments

Weight

For some women, the prospect of gaining weight whilst taking HRT is a real anxiety. Being weighed on the same (hopefully accurate) scales can be reassuring. For women who have a long-standing weight problem, it can be an ordeal to be weighed at each visit and is probably unnecessary in many instances. Being overweight will not, in itself, be a reason to tell a woman to stop her HRT. Measurement of weight is performed as a general health check rather than because the decision to continue HRT rests on the outcome, so you need to be sensitive to all women and think before you routinely weigh all women at every visit.

If a woman does gain weight whilst taking HRT, it is worth trying to establish whether it is cyclical (i.e. progestogen related), in which case that component of the therapy can be changed. Some apparent bloatedness may occur with the use of HRT, but this is most likely to be demonstrated by a tightening of rings or the waistband rather than a noticeable weight gain. A change of treatment may resolve this. For some women, the feeling of weight gain may be a reflection of fuller breasts and a return to a more normal female fat distribution, i.e. around the hips and thighs rather than the abdomen.

Blood pressure

It has become established practice to record the blood pressure of women who take HRT, yet there is no good evidence that blood pressure will be altered simply by the use of HRT (Utian 1978, Wren & Routledge 1983). Women who gain weight may see a rise in blood pressure. If hypertension is detected while a woman is taking HRT, she will need assessment and treatment for her blood pressure in its own right.

Symptom assessment

It is helpful for a woman to review her symptoms once she is settled on HRT. Some symptoms may have disappeared, others may be improving and yet others may not have been affected at all. A symptom assessment score can help a woman to recognize those symptoms that may have decreased in intensity, even though they have not disappeared altogether. A chart will also help you to raise those symptoms that the woman may be embarrassed to discuss, yet which could be troublesome, for instance, bladder symptoms or sexual concerns. It can also be reassuring for a woman to be able to look back at a previous chart and recognize how much she has improved, perhaps without even realizing at the time. Occasionally an increase in dose will be necessary to further improve general symptoms.

Side-effects

If a woman has received adequate information before starting HRT, she will hopefully have reached her initial assessment visit without stopping treatment. By this time, side-effects should be diminishing and a more accurate assessment of the suitability of her HRT will be possible. If she is still experiencing side-effects, a change of HRT may be required.

It is important to try to establish, by direct questioning, when side-effects occur. Oestrogen-related side-effects are often continuous and may be relieved by adjusting the dose or changing the type or route of oestrogen. Progestogenic effects often persist for as long as that particular progestogen is taken; again, a change in dose or type of progestogen may be needed. There are established doses of progestogen that are considered to offer endometrial protection, and few doctors will recommend a lower dose than this, except in unusual circumstances. The duration of cyclical progestogen is also unlikely to be altered except by a specialist, but sometimes changing to a different progestogen is sufficient to reduce unwanted effects.

In cases of severe progestogenic side-effects and under the guidance of a specialist, it may be suggested that more radical steps be taken, such as prescribing oestrogen alone or even offering a hysterectomy. These are controversial issues and decisions that are likely to be made by a specialist who can offer the necessary support and follow-up that may be necessary.

Some women experience so-called side-effects, which are minor but troublesome. These can often be resolved if the woman is given the opportunity to express them. Often, they relate to the practicalities of taking the medication, for example patches that persistently fall off or cause a minor irritation may be a result of a woman not using them correctly. For instance, she may be applying the patch to wet skin or over talcum powder, not realizing that this will affect how well they stick.

Withdrawal bleed

At each follow-up visit, a woman taking a cyclical regimen of HRT should be asked directly about her withdrawal bleed. It is important because, if the bleed is abnormal, it could be a sign that the dose of HRT needs adjusting. It is also good to find out whether the bleed is what you would normally expect with use of HRT and whether it is acceptable to the woman herself. You should discuss the following issues.

Timing. Does the bleed occur at the approximate time you would expect it for the regimen she is taking? It is normal for the bleed to start at, or near, the end of the course of progestogen or a couple of days later. Erratic bleeding is common during the early stages of so-called 'period free' HRT.

Intensity. The bleed should not be unacceptably heavy and is normally similar to or lighter than a normal period. Some women will experience only a very light bleed or even no bleeding at all. This is considered normal, although some specialists would recommend that ultrasonography be performed, showing endometrial thickness. An over-thickened endometrium (greater than 4 mm after a progestogen phase) indicates the need for further investigation to ensure that safety of the endometrium is being maintained. A change of progestogen may be necessary. You should also check that the regimen is being taken correctly and that the progestogen is not being missed, either through error or intentionally.

Duration. Withdrawal bleeds commonly last up to 7 days, with many women experiencing bleeding for only 2 or 3 days, once they are established on treatment.

Irregular bleeding. You should ask whether any extra bleeding has occurred outside the normal monthly bleed (Fig. 7.3). Mid-cycle bleeding on a regular basis or postcoital bleeding should be investigated. Occasional irregular bleeding could be caused by concurrent medications such as antibiotics, or by a stomach upset causing a disturbance in absorption. Poor compliance could also be a cause. If you consider that the bleed is not as it should be, the woman would need to see the doctor with a view to a change of treatment or further investigation.

Breast examination

In 1998, the Department of Health recommended that doctors and nurses should no longer perform routine breast palpation (DoH 1998a). The question arises whether women on HRT fall into the category of 'routine' or into a 'high risk' group because of their HRT use. Physicians who believe the latter advocate annual breast checks as a precaution. However, even if breast examinations were carried out annually on all women using HRT, there would still be

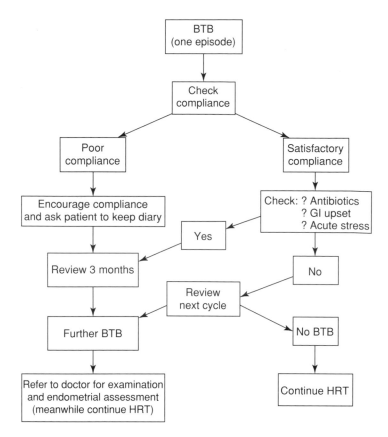

Figure 7.3 Guidelines for the management of breakthrough bleeding. BTB, breakthrough bleeding; GI, gastrointestinal.

no guarantee that any extra cases of breast cancer would be identified as the majority of breast cancers are identified by women themselves (DoH 1998a). It is more important to promote breast awareness. The Department of Health five-point code of breast awareness (DoH 1998b) states that women should:

◆ know what is normal for them
◆ become familiar with the look and feel of their own breasts
◆ know what changes to look for
◆ report any changes without delay
◆ attend for breast screening if aged 50 years or over.

Pelvic examination

There is no need for extra routine pelvic examinations just because a woman is taking HRT (Page & Glasier 2000). Some specialists ensure that one is performed 3 yearly along with cervical cytology. Occasionally, there will be a clinical indication for an extra examination, and you may need to refer the woman to the doctor in these instances (Box 7.3).

Question time

When a woman returns to clinic for a routine follow-up, there is a tendency to carry out the necessary procedures, ask the relevant questions and move on to the next patient. HRT is a medication that is not usually being taken for a life-threatening disease, and monitoring a woman on therapy can appear very routine. Women may have questions that they want to ask, but often feel that the opportunity to do so does not present itself. Women may wish to discuss whether to come off treatment or may have minor anxieties that could be easily allayed. It is therefore helpful to make a point of asking each woman whether there are any issues she would like to discuss. Opportunity is then given for women to ask questions that, in themselves, are probably not medically important but that, once answered, enable the woman to feel more confident about her treatment. Such issues may include:

◆ media coverage of HRT
◆ underlying anxieties about breast cancer
◆ advice received from 'friends'

Box 7.3 Indications for extra pelvic examination

◆ Postcoital bleeding
◆ Irregular bleeding
◆ Pelvic pain
◆ Episodes of intermenstrual bleeding

◆ practical issues about taking her HRT
◆ advice about alternative therapy options.

Nurse or doctor?

In the past, women on HRT expected to see a doctor regularly for monitoring and assessment. Now that practice nurses are becoming much more involved in the care and assessment of all patients, it is common for them to be doing some of the monitoring of treatment (Fig. 7.3). In the same way that nurses are trained in contraception and sexual health care for women on the contraceptive pill, suitably trained nurses could do much of the routine monitoring of HRT. As well as releasing the time for their doctor colleagues, it will more importantly lead to a 'team approach' in caring for women at the time of the menopause. Many women will be pleased to have the opportunity to see the nurse rather than the doctor on some occasions, particularly as it is not uncommon for them to have longer (more realistic) appointment times, which are more conducive to discussion (Quantock & Beynon 1995).

As with all areas of medicine, it is important that nurses recognize their abilities and establish guidelines as to when referral back to a doctor is necessary. It is useful to have a protocol agreed by doctors and nurses within a team, so that all staff involved are working to agreed and consistent standards of care (see Ch. 9).

When to refer to a doctor
◆ Poorly controlled symptoms
◆ Unmanageable or unexpected side-effects
◆ On discovery of a breast lump
◆ Abnormal bleeding pattern
◆ At a woman's own request.

SUMMARY

The menopause can seem like a life-changing event to some women. The opportunity to discuss issues and learn about different therapy options is often gratefully appreciated. The assessment of a woman before starting HRT and the ongoing monitoring thereafter is satisfying work. Many women present with a number of prob lems, sometimes unable to clarify for themselves which are hormone related and which are not. Spending time with such women is time well spent and women themselves are often very grateful for the help and advice they receive. Time spent advising a woman before she starts treatment may save time later, and also ensures that the woman is in a position to make a truly informed choice about HRT. Preparing women fully for HRT will result in them having realistic expectations and subsequently be less likely to stop treatment after only a short while. This is particularly relevant to women considering long-term HRT.

REFERENCES

Andersson K, Pederson AT, Mattson L, Milsom L (1998) Swedish gynaecologists' and GPs' views on the climacteric period: knowledge, attitudes and management strategies. *Acta Obstet. Gynecol. Scand.* **77**: 909–916.

Department of Health (1998a) *Clinical Examination of the Breast.* PL/CMO/98. DoH, London.

Department of Health (1998b) *Be Breast Aware.* K6L/006 14343 PDD 50K 2P. DoH, London.

Hall G, Spector TD (1992) Hormone replacement therapy – why do so few women use it? *Osteoporosis Rev.* **1**: 2.

Karakoc B, Erenus M (1998) Compliance considerations with HRT. *Menopause* **5**: 102–106.

Newton KM, La Croix AZ, Levelle SG et al (1997) Women's beliefs and decisions about HRT. *J Womens Health* **6**: 459–465.

Page C, Glasier A (2000) Monitoring of HRT – what should we be doing? In: Studd JW (ed.) *The Management of the Menopause, Millenium Review,* pp. 49–58. Parthenon, London.

Quantock C, Beynon J (1995) HRT and the nurse counsellor. *Nursing Standard* **9**: (40): 20–21.

Royal College of Radiologists Working Party (1998) *Making the Best Use of Clinical Radiology: Guidelines for Doctors,* 4th edn. RCR, London.

Rymer JM (1998) The effects of tibolone. *Gynecol. Endocrinol.* **12**: 213–220.

Ulrich LG, Barlow DH, Sturdee DW et al (1997) Quality of life and patient preference for sequential versus continuous combined HRT: the Kliofem multicentre study experience. *Int. J. Gynaecol. Obstet.* **59** (Suppl 1): S11–17.

Utian W (1978) Effect of postmenopausal oestrogen therapy on diastolic blood pressure and body weight. *Maturitas* **1**: 3.

Wren BG, Routledge AD (1983) The effect of type and dose of oestrogen on the blood pressure of postmenopausal women. *Maturitas* **5**: 135–142.

Non-hormonal Methods for Coping with Menopausal Symptoms

Denise Tiran

INTRODUCTION

The menopause is a natural physiological life event that affects all women in later life. Some women sail through the perimenopausal stage with no real problems, whereas others experience a range of symptoms which may cause them concern, discomfort or inconvenience at some time. Some women may require medically prescribed treatments to help them cope, but others may feel disempowered by medical intervention and wish to try other, more natural, methods to relieve their symptoms. This is characteristic of a general trend in healthcare access, for many people feel disenchanted with and distrustful of the medical professions, which are not always able to fulfil the demands of the service.

Partly in response to this, complementary and alternative medicine (CAM) is a growing area of health care which is increasingly being recognized and accepted by the general public and by practitioners of conventional health care (Yardley & Furnham 1999). Women may have used complementary therapies previously for themselves or their families, either for relaxation and general well-being, or for more specific clinical conditions to enhance orthodox management. It is thought that about a third of the population in the UK has consulted a practitioner of complementary medicine (Stone 1999), and in the USA this may be as high as 1 in 2.

Fundamental to the provision of CAM therapies is the focus on individualizing care in order to treat the whole person, rather than merely the disease or condition. Whole-person medicine is based on the concept of body–mind–spirit, and practitioners believe it is vital to take all three aspects into account. A pathological condition may be exacerbated by emotional or spiritual factors, or vice versa. It is suggested that the very fact that the menopause is a normal life event lends itself to management using a holistic framework, rather than focusing on a biological framework or a psychosocial model, which can stigmatize the essential female condition whilst omitting other essential factors (Ulacia et al 1999).

CAM therapies are gradually becoming more integrated into orthodox care, especially in the primary care setting, although increasingly also in secondary and tertiary care. The British Medical Association (1993) acknowledged that certain elements of CAM were of benefit to patients and clients. The Foundation for Integrated Medicine (FIM), a charity established to promote further integration of the therapies into conventional health care, made recommendations regarding the education and training of health-care professionals using these therapies, whether primarily complementary or conventional practitioners (FIM 1997). FIM also expressed concern about regulation of the many different therapies, as well as the evidence base required to facilitate further integration into orthodox healthcare systems. There are well over 200 complementary and alternative therapies, although in reality only about 20 are currently considered to be credible and acceptable. In 2000, the House of Lords Select Committee on Science and Technology published its sixth report, on complementary medicine, reclassifying the numerous therapies into three main groups (see Box 8.1) and making recommendations for safe accountable practice.

Box 8.1 Classification of complementary and alternative therapies according to the sixth report of the House of Lords Select Committee on Science and Technology (2000)

Group 1

Therapies that have a reasonable scientific body of evidence of effectiveness, are professionally organized with approved methods of education for practitioners, and are discrete systems of health care in their own right:

◆ homeopathy

◆ acupuncture

◆ osteopathy

◆ chiropractic

◆ herbal medicine.

Group 2

Therapies that lack any real scientific basis and are not yet regulated nationally but which give comfort and support to many people:

◆ aromatherapy

◆ reflexology

◆ massage

◆ Bach flower remedies

◆ nutritional therapy

◆ hypnotherapy

◆ yoga

◆ shiatsu

◆ Alexander technique

◆ counselling and stress management.

Box 8.1 (*Contd.*)

Group 3
Therapies that are alternative to conventional health care with no established body of evidence to support claims of efficacy and safety including Traditional Chinese Medicine, Ayurvedic medicine, anthroposophical medicine, naturopathy, crystal therapy, kinesiology, radionics, dowsing and iridology.
It is not the intention of this chapter to cover these therapies. More information can be found in the References and the Appendix.

THE NURSE AND COMPLEMENTARY AND ALTERNATIVE THERAPIES

Nurses who come into contact with women seeking alternatives to HRT should be mindful of their own position and should refrain from giving advice unless they have been trained to do so. It is not necessary to be a fully qualified practitioner of a complementary therapy, but nurses, regulated by the UK Central Council for Nursing, Midwifery and Health Visiting (UKCC), should adhere to their professional Code of Conduct and Guidelines for Professional Practice (UKCC 1992, 1996). They should act always in the best interests of their patients, be able to justify their actions, and should ensure that the advice they give is based on currently available evidence and in accordance with health policies. It is not acceptable for nurses to 'dabble', *thinking* that they know what they are doing, without having received adequate and appropriate education on the subject. An example of this might be providing information to women on St John's wort, an increasingly recognized herbal antidepressant, of which many nurses will have heard. However, it is also essential to be aware of the Department of Health's paper sent out to all relevant health professionals (DoH 2000). This advised against recommending St John's wort to women taking the contraceptive pill, during pregnancy or breastfeeding, on anticoagulants, some cardiac and epileptic medications, and pharmacological antidepressants. This is because it is thought that the herbal remedy may inactivate or potentiate the action of certain drugs, and its use in pregnancy is unknown.

It is important, therefore, for readers to acknowledge that this chapter is intended as a means of raising awareness of natural alternatives to hormone replacement therapy (HRT). Many women will ask about them, but, as a general principle, women should be referred to an appropriately qualified and experienced complementary practitioner who also has a through understanding of the pathophysiology of the menopause. If a woman wishes to self-administer natural remedies such as herbal, aromatherapy or homeopathic substances, the nurse should facilitate this in the safest and most appropriate manner, whilst acknowledging the woman's right to do so.

AN INTRODUCTION TO THE MOST COMMONLY USED THERAPIES

Homeopathy

Homeopathy uses minute doses of substances derived from plants, minerals or, occasionally, animals, which, if given in large doses, would actually cause the problem that the practitioner is attempting to treat. Although many of the substances are administered in tablet form, as well as tinctures, creams or granules, they do not work pharmacologically, but are thought instead to work on the principles of vibrational energies.

Homeopathic remedies do not interfere with conventional medications but, in some instances, may be inactivated by them or by strong-smelling substances such as essential oils, peppermint or coffee. It is not true to say, however – despite the minute doses used – that homeopathic remedies are harmless. Like all complementary therapies, if they are powerful enough to act therapeutically, they may, if used inappropriately or inaccurately, either by error or intent, be potentially harmful

Homeopathic prescriptions are tailored to the *exact* nature of the individual's symptoms and take into account the personality and reactions of the person. Nurses should therefore be cautious when advocating homeopathic remedies to their patients. Examples given in this chapter are merely to illustrate the potential use of the remedies.

Bach flower remedies

A related therapy (group 2) which uses homeopathic principles is Bach flower remedies (BFRs), liquid preparations from a range of 38 plants which are designed to treat the emotional factors associated with illness or disease. The most popular of these is Rescue Remedy, readily available in health food stores and large pharmacies, and excellent for treating stress, shock, panic, nerves and hysteria. The dose is 4 drops neat on the tongue or in a small glass of water, as required. Doses of other BFRs are 2 drops in water, usually up to four times daily. Women can self-prescribe these with help from the literature available in the shops.

Acupuncture and acupressure

These are elements of Traditional Chinese Medicine (TCM), which is based on the use of 365 meridians, or energy lines, that run through the body from top to toe, passing through major organs, after which the 12 main meridians take their names. When the body, mind and spirit are in equilibrium, the energy (Chi) flowing along the meridians does so without impediment, but when disease is present blockages occur at specific points on the meridians (acupuncture points or *tsubos*). Inserting needles (acupuncture) or applying pressure (acupressure) to the points unblocks the energy and allows it to flow freely again.

A therapy similar to acupressure, which originated in Japan in the mid twentieth century, is *shiatsu* (group 2), which quite literally means 'thumb pressure' and incorporates a variety of massage techniques. Many people attend regularly for shiatsu massage as a means of maintaining well-being, although it can also be used to treat specific problems. It is interesting to note that acupuncture, frequently used in a reductionist, westernized manner by doctors, was classified by the House of Lords report (2000) into group 1, shiatsu is in group 2, while TCM has been relegated to group 3. Some elements of TCM, however, are discussed in the section on application to caring for women going through the menopause, for aspects such as **Tai Chi** and **Qi Gong**, based on original Chinese martial arts, are popularly available around the country as exercise and relaxation classes.

Osteopathy and chiropractic

These are related therapies involving manipulation of the musculoskeletal system in order to correct misalignments that may be causing tensions leading to illness or disease. Commonly people attend for musculoskeletal problems, but either therapy will be effective in treating soft tissue conditions such as duodenal ulcer or hiatus hernia. Osteopathy became statutorily regulated in 1993 and chiropractic followed in 1994; both are now considered to be professions supplementary to medicine rather than 'alternative' therapies. Osteopathy uses more massage and soft tissue manipulation than chiropractic, which works more directly on an affected area, but many of the principles are similar in both therapies. Chiropractic is the third most used system of health care in the world after conventional medicine and dentistry.

Herbal medicine

Herbal medicine is the precursor of modern pharmaceuticals, the original 'witchcraft', but is enjoying a resurgence of popularity due to dissatisfaction of the general public with the side-effects and complications of conventional drugs. Therapeutic agents derived from plants may be given in tablet, tincture, cream or liquid form (as teas) but all work pharmacologically, being absorbed, utilized, metabolized by and excreted from the body in the same way as drugs.

The difference between herbal remedies and drugs is that, if used correctly, the incidence of side-effects is much reduced with plant medicines. Often there are chemical constituents within the plant that balance and counteract the negative effects produced by the required active ingredient when it is isolated and synthesized in order for a pharmaceutical company to patent the product. An example of this is salicylate, found in willow bark, which when commercially produced as aspirin may cause gastritis, but when used by herbalists as an analgesic or anti-inflammatory in the context of the whole plant, does not. As with other therapies that are readily available over the counter, herbal medicine should not automatically be considered safe without question.

Aromatherapy

Aromatherapy is one element of herbal medicine, focusing specifically on the use of concentrated essential oils found in the cells of plants and harnessed for their therapeutic properties, which result from the chemical constituents within the oils (Fig. 8.1). Although the aromas are usually pleasant, the term 'aromatherapy' detracts from the highly scientific pharmacological means by which essential oils work. This is commonly compounded by the emphasis on the 'feel good' factor that comes from the method of administration of the oils, usually via massage, in the bath, by inhalation or in creams. Essential oils can also be administered in pessaries, suppositories or by mouth, although the latter should generally not be advocated to patients unless prescribed by a medically qualified doctor, as there is currently little available knowledge about the means and rate of metabolism when ingested.

In common with other therapies, aromatherapy is invaluable when used appropriately, but the ready accessibility to the general public has led to people believing that the oils are harmless, which is not necessarily true. For example, there are many essential oils that should not be used by people with hypertension, epilepsy, during pregnancy or with skin sensitivity. Doses must be kept as low as is therapeutically adequate, and good-quality uncontaminated oils used. They should be bought from reputable suppliers willing to provide chromatography analysis results if requested; popular

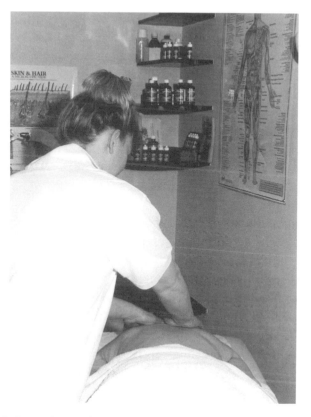

Figure 8.1 Aromatherapy. Reproduced with permission of Alison Campbell, beauty therapist. Photo by Mark Anernethy.

high-street shops do not always sell essential oils suitable for clinical practice and women should be discouraged from using these. Nurses should be careful to advise women about specific dangers of any oils they may wish to use: this can only come from an *in-depth* knowledge of the chemical constituents, pharmacological properties, side-effects and contraindications.

Reflexology

Reflexology is a sophisticated form of foot (or hand) manipulation in which the feet represent a map of the rest of the body so that every part of the body is reflected on one or both feet. By working on the specific areas of the feet, various health-related conditions can be treated, although the therapy is also invaluable as a relaxing method of boosting well-being. In keeping with other therapies, it is, however, not without danger if used inappropriately: it is possible to 'overdose' someone with reflexology or to exacerbate a condition through using the wrong technique. Reflexology is *not* simply foot massage, and nurses should ensure that women wishing to receive treatment consult a practitioner who is fully cognisant of their particular health needs.

Massage

Massage is the therapeutically applied use of touch in order to relax or, on occasions, to stimulate the body, mind and spirit. Massage assists in stimulating the circulation and excretory processes, relaxing joints and muscles, and inducing a feeling of relaxation and well-being. There are some contraindications to specific types of massage, such as avoiding varicosed areas or precise locations of tumours. There are many different forms of massage, including Swedish, lymphatic drainage, rolfing, Lomi-Lomi (Hawaiian) and others.

Nutritional therapy

Nutritional therapy is more than dietetics. Practitioners not only aim to assist people to adapt their diets according to their needs, but also seek to rebalance the nutritional status of the patient. They do this by examining the quality and quantity of food ingested, its metabolism, utilization, and excretion, and advocating the use of vitamin and mineral supplements to redress imbalances caused by diet, lifestyle and environmental factors.

Hypnotherapy

Hypnotherapy is the applied use of hypnosis for medical purposes, using a variety of deep relaxation techniques to aid psychological comfort. It is especially useful for altering the perception of pain and for changing habitual behaviour. Counselling plays a part, and medical hypnotherapists should be qualified counsellors. Contrary to popular opinion it is not possible to induce people to do things they have no wish to do, and it is unfortunate that the media has seen fit to ridicule some aspects of the therapy.

Yoga

Yoga is a disciplined form of exercise and posture, breathing and meditation which tones the body, aids suppleness, flexibility and strength, oxygenates the circulation and relaxes the mind. There are four different types of yoga, with most of those that are unspecified being hatha yoga, which is the most basic. Ashtanga yoga involves running postures and the building up of heat until sweating occurs, Iyengar yoga is a very precise form in which postures are practised separately, and Sivananda yoga incorporates diet and meditation as well as the physical component.

Alexander technique

This is a means of postural re-education in order to reduce or eliminate the discomfort and dis-ease that develops as a result of habitual poor use of the body. It originated when Alexander, an actor, discovered that throat tensions that were triggered by stage fright could be alleviated by improved posture; he went on to develop a system that is still used by actors today, as well as by many other people, to correct a range of disorders. Usually a series of classes, mostly on a one-to-one basis, is required, but for many use of the Alexander technique becomes a way of life.

USING COMPLEMENTARY AND ALTERNATIVE THERAPIES FOR SPECIFIC SYMPTOMS DURING THE CLIMACTERIC PHASE

Anxiety, irritability and mood changes

Mood changes, irritability, aggression and food cravings can occur at times of hormonal fluctuations as a result of low blood sugar levels; therefore, maintaining a consistent level is important to prevent such symptoms. Certain substances, such as the stimulants of tea, coffee, cola, sugar and alcohol, cause a rise in the level of blood sugar which is followed by a sharp fall as the sugars are readily metabolized. This leads to a rise in adrenaline as the body seeks to correct the imbalance and, even without the trigger of external stressors, responds as if stressed, producing feelings of anxiety and tension. Women should be advised to eat little and often, and to avoid foods that are high in sugars or stimulants. Complex carbohydrates and foods such as bananas will have longer-lasting effects in stabilizing the blood sugar levels. Added to this the nutrients that are considered to be calming should be advised, such as foods containing vitamin B complex and magnesium, or women may benefit from a daily supplement of these.

Nervine plants, those that act as antidepressants and relaxants, may be appropriate herbal remedies. Skullcap, combined with valerian, is sometimes prescribed by qualified therapists, while ginseng is a tonic aimed at reducing anxiety. Ginseng is an adaptogen which has a balancing effect on the body and mind. St John's wort is a herbal preparation of *Hypericum perforatum* which has been well researched in Germany and other countries. Its use is as an antidepressant, and it is thought to work by inhibiting serotonin uptake by increasing the concentration of sodium ions (Nathan 1999, Singer et al 1999), although Deltito & Beyer (1998) recommend its use only in cases of mild to moderate depression. Mood swings and hormonal tension and anxiety also respond to Vitex agnus castus. Lauritzen et al's study (1997) into premenstrual tension may usefully be applied to the care of perimenopausal women as Vitex agnus castus showed a reduction in depression, stress and anxiety, although side-effects were demonstrated in a small proportion of women.

Some aromatherapy oils may be useful, either as a means of general relaxation (e.g. lavender) or for uplifting the mood (e.g. bergamot). Research has shown that jasmine has a more calming effect than was previously thought (Imberger et al 1993, Karamat et al

1992). The method of administration may have some effect, with massage being the most relaxing, but women could also add 4 drops of the oils, in a good-quality carrier oil such as sweet almond, to their baths. Other generally relaxing therapies include shiatsu, reflexology and hypnotherapy, as well as more active forms of relaxation such as Tai Chi, Qi Gong or yoga. Hypnotherapy may assist women psychologically in coming to terms with the changes of the climacteric, especially when compounded by other concerns such as obesity (Allison & Faith 1996, Stradling et al 1998), which may deal indirectly with feelings of anxiety or depression. Although there is no research evidence to support their use, Bach flower remedies can usefully be self-administered, including larch for low self-confidence and self-esteem, mustard for dejection, and walnut to help the woman adapt to change.

Breast tenderness and discomfort

Vitex agnus castus is thought to balance female hormones, especially oestrogens, and as well as relieving psychological complaints has been shown to reduce breast tenderness (Lauritzen et al 1997). In Chinese medicine it is thought that breast tenderness and 'lumpy' breasts are a sign of inadequate Liver energy (Chi) and may, in Western terms, indicate poor metabolism by the liver of the oestrogens that are fluctuating in concentration within the body at the time of the menopause. Therefore, many therapies aim to detoxify the liver, either with herbs such as dandelion and milk thistle, or through acupuncture, shiatsu or reflexology. It is pertinent here to comment on the fact that phytoestrogens (plant oestrogens), often used by women to reduce symptoms such as flushes (see below), have been queried in relation to possible breast cancer, but recent debate suggests that ingestion in early life of plants known to contain oestrogen-like substances may have a protective effect (Barnes 1998, Bingham et al 1998, Lu & Anderson 1998, Stephens 1999).

Metabolism of excess oestrogens is also the theory behind using nutritional supplements such as vitamin B complex to assist the liver in inactivating oestrogen no longer required. Vitamin B_6 is a particularly beneficial supplement, while *Lactobacillus acidophilus*, found in live natural yogurt or taken as capsules, lowers the enzymes that reabsorb 'old' oestrogens (Glenville 1997). Essential oils such as cypress or juniper berry are thought to relieve excess fluid, although the latter should be avoided in women with renal problems. Reflexology may ease some of the discomfort; it has been shown to alleviate breast tenderness in the premenstrual phase when performed regularly (Oleson & Flocco 1993).

Headaches and migraine

Many women experience hormonally induced headaches and migraine, and head massage may be helpful for some. Touch impulses reach the brain before pain impulses, and deep scalp massage will often also focus on relevant acupressure points. Migraine sufferers who receive massage have been shown to have increased levels of serotonin and a reduction in the number and severity of attacks (Hernandez Reif et al 1998).

Reflex zone therapy to the foot zones for the head, neck and shoulders is not only relaxing but can also work specifically on the affected areas. A comparison between reflex zone therapy and a standard pharmaceutical preparation used to treat headache showed no significant difference in the degree of analgesia, or in the time taken for the patient to obtain relief, but a lower incidence of side-effects was found in the reflex zone therapy group (Eichelberger 1993). Applying 2 drops of neat lavender essential oil to the temples can be sufficient in some cases, or may work synergistically if used with peppermint oil. Practitioners of herbal medicine may prescribe dandelion, milk thistle or feverfew, although the latter is best taken regularly as a preventive rather than at the time of a migraine. Vitex agnus castus may help (Lauritzen et al 1997).

Acupuncture will work on the relevant meridians, such as the Liver meridian, as headaches may be a sign of depleted Liver energy (Chi). Osteopathy or chiropractic can realign neck and spinal tensions, so relaxing the neck and head, and may help to improve hormonal functioning by reducing tensions in the areas of pertinent glands. Similarly, the Alexander technique can realign the woman's posture to alleviate head and neck pain made worse by cervical vertebral tensions.

Tiredness, lack of energy and insomnia

One of the simplest instant remedies for tiredness and lethargy is the Bach flower remedy, Olive. Two drops, neat, placed on the tongue may be sufficient to enable a woman to continue with her day, although it is not a substitute for adequate sleep and rest. The typical 'Monday morning' feeling can be overcome with hornbeam, another of the BFR range.

Certain nutrients may boost energy levels, whereas other foods may reduce them. Sugar and stimulants may offer a 'quick fix' but are usually counterproductive in the longer term and are best reduced or eliminated altogether. Coenzyme Q10, a substance present in all organs, increases energy production, but the ageing process decreases the ability to produce Q10 naturally from the food eaten, so supplements may be helpful. Other nutrients include the vitamin B complex, although this should be taken early in the day to avoid restlessness at night, and iron-containing foods to prevent anaemia. Magnesium supplements may act as a natural tranquillizer. Herbal ginseng may also assist in increasing energy levels, but women should not rely on this consistently.

Insomnia can be aided by encouraging women to practise relaxation exercises. Adequate exercise during the day will boost endorphin levels and facilitate better-quality natural sleep. Two drops of lavender oil neat on the pillow can be inhaled and may induce deeper relaxation, or the essential oil may be added to the bath. It is not a good idea to advise the use of burners and vaporizers at night, partly for safety reasons, but also because the maximum number of molecules that the human nose can absorb will be reached within 10 minutes. Leaving a vaporizer on for longer than this can lead to nausea and headaches (for both the woman and any partner).

Massage, reflexology or shiatsu on a regular basis can enhance relaxation and, if performed in the evening, may induce sleep. Hynotherapy may be helpful for some women.

If insomnia is exacerbated by constant thoughts – the mind going over and over things and being unable to 'switch off' – homeopathic coffea may be the most appropriate remedy, whilst others are more appropriate when the symptoms differ. Herbal valerian or passiflora (passion flower) are useful remedies to aid the onset of sleep and can be bought in a commercially available form. The alkaloids contained in passiflora are thought to work directly on the central nervous system to induce sleep. The advantage of herbal sleeping tablets is that they do not produce the lethargy and 'hungover' feeling that may occur with some pharmaceutical sedatives.

Hot flushes and sweating

Osteopathy or chiropractic may be of use in rebalancing some of the hormonal fluctuations that lead to hot flushes, particularly when minor, previously insignificant, musculoskeletal misalignments cause tensions, especially in the cervical vertebrae, which may put undue strain on the pituitary gland (Wallis 1994).

Similarly, acupuncture has been found to reduce the incidence and severity of intermittent hot flushes in some women (Wyon et al 1995). Homeopathic remedies may include capsicum (sweet pepper) or, if accompanied by mood changes and headaches or migraine, amyl nitrosum. Other women with hot flushes who also experience cravings for sweet foods and alcohol, and who have profuse sweating which triggers periods of being argumentative, may respond to sulfur (Katz 1997). A proprietary homeopathic remedy, Feminon N, has been found by Polish researchers to relieve some menopausal symptoms, including hot flushes, and to reduce levels of follicle stimulating hormone, but not oestradiol (Warenik-Szymankiewicz et al 1997).

Herbal Vitex agnus castus appears to be particularly effective in relieving hot flushes and night sweats, and yarrow, a plant long known for its antipyrexial action, may also help.

Phytoestrogens, plants that contain weakly oestrogenic constituents, have been investigated in relation to menopausal symptoms in recent years. Eden (1998) suggests that hot flushes may be helped by increasing the amount of phytoestrogens in the daily diet, although they do not seem to have a beneficial effect in dealing with vaginal dryness. Whitten & Natfolin (1998) examined the value of phytoestrogens for a range of symptoms as HRT alternatives, while Scheiber & Rebar (1999) advocated further trials. In nutritional therapy, bioflavonoids combined with vitamin C are thought to reduce hot flushes more effectively than HRT, possibly by toning the blood vessels and thereby preventing excessive vasodilatation and consequent sweating, a process normally achieved by circulating oestrogens (Glenville 1997).

Aromatherapy essential oils that may assist in reducing the impact of hot flushes include Roman chamomile, although this has not been proven. Black pepper oil is considered to be a warming oil and may, if used almost in homeopathic dilution, relieve sweats and flushes.

Natural progesterone cream, derived from the wild yam, has been widely publicized to women as an effective treatment for hot flushes, but to date there have been no randomized controlled studies to support its use. Such trials are underway and the results are awaited with interest.

Dysmenorrhoea and menorrhagia

Excessive menstrual bleeding may be treated by homeopathy using, for example, murex, if accompanied by depression and a raised libido (Katz 1997). If fibroids are found to be partly the cause and hysterectomy is recommended, arnica for bruising and hypericum for wound healing may be useful homeopathic remedies, although research has not produced any conclusive evidence of this (Ernst & Pittler 1998, Hart et al 1997, Linde et al 1997, Vickers et al 1998).

Menorrhagia and dysmenorrhoea appear to be associated with an increase in the production of series 2 prostaglandins, possibly exacerbated by an increase in arachidonic acid, which is found in milk, meat and some essential fatty acids such as linseed. It therefore follows that reducing the consumption of these foodstuffs may assist in controlling the symptoms (Glenville 1997). Obviously steps must also be taken to prevent anaemia both by increasing iron-containing foods and those rich in vitamin C to enhance uptake, as well as eliminating from the diet substances that inhibit iron absorption, such as tea. Acupuncture or shiatsu may assist in rebalancing hormone output.

If dysmenorrhoea becomes a problem, certain shiatsu techniques may be used to alleviate back and suprapubic pain, or compresses of clary sage essential oil can be applied, or the oil added to the bath water. Geranium oil is thought to be a hormone balancer, and Roman chamomile is antispasmodic owing to the presence of high levels of esters (Price 1993, Rossi et al 1988). Herbal products such as cramp bark, as its name suggests, are well known to relieve menstrual cramping, having constituents that are antispasmodic and muscle relaxing. Skullcap and black cohosh are also beneficial. Reflexology can be used both as a general relaxing treatment and to relieve specific pain.

Poor concentration and memory loss

Women should be encouraged to remain mentally active, perhaps taking up new studies, such as attending evening classes, in order that mental agility, memory and concentration are retained. Preventing atherosclerosis of cerebral vessels, as well as others, can be assisted by advising a reduction in saturated fats in the diet and increasing fruit and vegetable content to at least five portions daily. Vitamin and mineral supplements of B_6, E and C, magnesium and selenium, or a good multivitamin, will enhance overall well-being. Ginkgo biloba, a herbal product, is thought to affect the brain positively, increasing cerebral circulation and assisting in cerebral energy by increasing glucose and oxygen supplies to the brain (Glenville 1997). Undertaking physical exercise encourages the brain to function, coordinating muscular activity and triggering serotonin production; therefore activities such as yoga, Tai Chi or Qi Gong may be helpful.

Bach flower remedies are useful for specific psychological problems which can sometimes cloud the mind and contribute to poor concentration; for example, walnut is particularly effective in helping adaptation to change. Clematis, honeysuckle or white chestnut may also be of help.

Vaginal dryness

Using herbal remedies to regulate hormonal function may assist in preventing this problem, or in lessening the effects. Motherwort is thought to improve the elasticity and thickness of the endometrium, and Chinese dong quai may help with lubrication for sexual intercourse. The changing pH of the vagina may also predispose the woman to vaginal infection such as thrush and, in this instance, essential oils come into their own. There are numerous clinical trials regarding the anti-infective properties of essential oils in general and of tea tree in particular, and commercial preparations of tea tree are also available in health food stores. It is, however, important that the tea tree (*Melaleuca alternifolia*) is designated 'terpineol-4-ol rich', as this has been found to be the most active ingredient (Altman 1989, Belaiche 1985, Carson & Riley 1995, Carson et al 1996, Pena 1962, Southwell et al 1997, Williams et al 1998, Zarno 1994). The use of vaginal moisturizers, such as Replens, is also useful.

Exercise that increases pelvic circulation can be encouraged, such as swimming and cycling; pelvic floor exercises will also improve blood supply to this area. Maintaining vaginal health will increase lubrication, leading to fewer problems with intercourse which, in itself, can stimulate endorphin production, so leading to improved overall well-being.

Mobility and prevention of osteoporosis

It is obviously important to encourage women to pursue some form of physical exercise, even simple walking, as this will facilitate the production of endorphins to aid mental relaxation, enhance the quality of sleep and encourage suppleness and mobility. Yoga classes may suit some and have been found to increase cardiovascular function (Peng et al 1999, Raju et al 1997, Schmidt et al 1997, Stachenfeld et al 1998) and improve manual dexterity (Manjunath & Telles 1999, Raghuraj & Telles 1997). Similarly, Tai Chi may reduce high blood pressure (Selvamurthy et al 1998), especially when combined with moderate aerobic exercise (Lai et al 1995, Young et al 1999), as well as enhancing general fitness (Lan et al 1998). Research has also demonstrated the positive effects on posture and balance in preventing falls in older women (Forrest 1997, Henderson et al 1998, Lane & Nydick 1999, Schaller 1996, Wolf et al 1996, Wolfson et al 1996).

Where problems such as backache prevent adequate exercise, osteopathy or chiropractic may be helpful in alleviating the condition (Giles and Muller 1999, Meade 1999). The effect on the opioid receptors of β-endorphins and neuropeptides makes acupuncture a possible alternative treatment for chronic pain or that caused by illnesses such as cancer (Andersson & Lundeberg 1995, Bin 1995, Bin et al 1994, Camp 1995, ter Riet et al 1990). Seidl & Stewart (1998) suggest that phytoestrogens may protect women from osteoporosis, as do Anderson & Garner (1998), although the latter point out that work has been carried out on postmenopausal women only in relation to the lumbar vertebrae.

CONCLUSION

The menopause is a natural life event which lends itself admirably to the use of natural remedies and therapies to help women deal with some of the symptoms and discomforts they experience. Nurses are in an invaluable position to advocate the safe effective use of some of these therapies, applying their knowledge of the physiology, contemporary conventional treatments and suitable alternatives to the care of women who consult them. Nurses must be mindful of their professional accountability in these circumstances and refrain from advising or doing anything that is outside the remit of their professional boundaries, or for which they have not been adequately trained. The very fact that women are often widely read and may know more about natural alternatives than the nurse makes it essential that health professionals are aware of sources of information and have ready access to research and authoritative information in order to assist their patients in the best possible manner.

REFERENCES

Allison DB, Faith MS (1996) Hypnosis as an adjunct to cognitive–behavioural psychotherapy for obesity: a meta-analysis reappraisal. *J. Consult. Clin. Psychol.* **64**(3): 513–516.

Altman PM (1989) Australian tea tree oil – a natural antiseptic. *Aust. J. Biotechnol.* **3**(4): 247–248.

Anderson JJ, Garner SC (1998) Phytoestrogens and bone. *Baillieres Clin. Endocrinol. Metab.* **12**(4): 527–543.

Andersson S, Lundeberg T (1995) Acupuncture: from empiricism to science – functional background to acupuncture effects in pain and disease. *Med. Hypotheses* **45**(3): 271.

Barnes S (1998) Phytoestrogens and breast cancer. *Baillieres Clin. Endocrinol. Metab.* **12**(4): 559–579.

Belaiche P (1985) Treatment of vaginal infections of *Candida albicans* with the essential oil of *Melaleuca alternifolia*. *Phyotherapy* **15**: 13–15.

Bin W (1995) Effect of acupuncture on the regulation of cell mediated immunity in patients with malignant tumours. *Chen Tzu Yen Chiu* **20**(3): 67.

Bin W, Zhou RX, Zhou MS (1994) Effect of acupuncture on interleukin-2 level and NK cell immunoactivity of peripheral blood of malignant tumour patients. *Chung Kuo His I Chieh Ho Tsa Chih* **14**(9): 537.

Bingham SA, Atkinson C, Liggins J et al (1998) Phyoestrogens – where are we now? *Br. J. Nutr.* **79**(5): 393–406.

British Medical Association (1993) *Complementary Medicine: New Approaches to Good Practice.* Oxford University Press, London.

Camp V (1995) The place of acupuncture in medicine today. *Br. J. Rheumatol.* **34**(5): 404.

Carson CF, Riley TV (1995) Antimicrobial activity of the major components of the essential oil of *Melaleuca alternifolia*. *J. Appl. Bacteriol.* **78**(3): 264–269.

Carson CF, Hammer KA, Riley TV (1996) In vitro activity of the essential oil of *Melaleuca alternifolia* against *Streptococcus* spp. *J. Antimicrob. Chemother.* **37**(6): 1177–1181.

Deltito J, Beyer D (1998) The scientific, quasi-scientific and popular literature on the use of St John's wort in the treatment of depression. *J. Affect. Dis.* **51**(3): 345–351.

Department of Health (2000) Guidelines on St John's wort. DoH, London.

Eden J (1998) Phytoestrogens and the menopause. *Baillieres Clin. Endocrinol. Metab.* **12**(4): 581–587.

Eichelberger G (1993) Studie uber Fussreflex-zonenmassage – Alternative zu Pillen. *Krankenpfl-Soins Infirm.* **86**(5): 61–63.

Ernst E, Pittler MH (1998) Efficacy of homeopathic arnica – a systematic review of placebo-controlled trials. *Arch. Surg.* **133**(11): 1187–1190.

Forrest WR (1997) Anticipatory postural adjustment and Tai Chi Chuan. *Biomed. Sci. Instrum.* **33**: 65–70.

Foundation for Integrated Medicine (1997) *Integrated Healthcare: A Way Forward for the Next Five Years?* FIM, London.

Giles LG, Muller R (1999) Chronic spinal pain syndromes: a clinical pilot trial comparing acupuncture, a non-steroidal anti-inflammatory drug and spinal manipulation. *J. Manipulative Physiol. Ther.* **22**(6): 376–381.

Glenville M (1997) *Natural Alternatives to HRT*. Kyle Cathie, London.

Hart O, Mullee MA, Lewith G, Miller J (1997) Double-blind placebo-controlled randomized clinical trial of homeopathic arnica 30C for pain and infection after total abdominal hysterectomy. *J. R. Soc. Med.* **90**(2): 73–78.

Henderson NK, White CP, Eisman JA (1998) The roles of exercise and fall risk reduction in the prevention of osteoporosis. *Endocrinol. Metab. Clin. North Am.* **27**(2): 369–387.

Hernandez Reif M, Dieter J, Field T et al (1998) Migraine headaches are reduced by massage therapy. *Int. J. Neurosci.* **96**(1–2): 1–11.

House of Lords Select Committee on Science and Technology (2000) *Sixth Report on Complementary and Alternative Medicine*. HMSO, London.

Imberger I, Rupp J, Karamat C, Buchbauer G (1993) Effects of essential oils on human attentional processes. 24th International Symposium on Essential Oils (abstract).

Karamat E, Imberger J, Buchbauer G et al (1992) Excitory and sedative effects of essential oils on human reaction time performance. *Chemical Senses* **17**: 847.

Katz T (1997) Homeopathic treatment during the menopause. *Complem. Ther. Nursing Midwif.* **3**(2): 46–50.

Lai JS, Lan C, Wong MK, Teng SH (1995) Two year trends in cardiorespiratory function among older Tai Chi Chuan practitioners and sedentary subjects. *J. Am. Geriatr. Soc.* **43**(11): 1222–1227.

Lan C, Lai JS, Chen SY, Wong MK (1998) 12 month Tai Chi training in the elderly: its effects on health fitness. *Med. Sci. Sports Exerc.* **30**(3): 345–351.

Lane JM, Nydick M (1999) Osteoporosis: current modes of prevention and treatment. *J. Am. Acad. Orthoped. Surg.* **7**(1): 19–31.

Lauritzen C, Reuter HD, Repges R et al (1997) Treatment of premenstrual tension syndrome with *Vitex agnus castus* – controlled double-blind study versus pyridoxine. *Phytomedicine* **4**(3): 183–189.

Linde K, Clausius N, Ramirez G et al (1997) Are the clinical effects of homeopathy placebo effects? A meta-analysis of placebo-controlled trials. *Lancet* **350**(9081): 834–843.

Lu LJ, Anderson KE (1998) Sex and longterm soy diets affect the metabolism and excretion of soy isoflavones in humans. *Am. J. Hum. Nutr.* **68**(6 Suppl): 1500S–1504S.

Manjunath NK, Telles S (1999) Factors influencing change in tweezer dexterity scores following yoga training. *Indian J. Physiol. Pharmacol.* **43**(2): 225–229.

Meade TW (1999) Patients are more satisfied with chiropractic than other treatments for low back pain. *Br. Med. J. (Clin. Res.)* **319**(7201): 57 (letter).

Nathan PJ (1999) The experimental and clinical pharmacology of St John's wort (*Hypericum perforatum* L.). *Mol. Psychiatry* **4**(4): 333–338.

Oleson T, Flocco W (1993) Randomized controlled study of premenstrual symptoms treated with ear, hand and foot reflexology. *Obstet. Gynecol.* **82**(6): 906–911.

Pena EF (1962) *Melaleuca alternifolia* oil. Its use for trichomonas vaginitis and other vaginal infections. *Obstet. Gynecol.* **19**(6): 793–795.

Peng CK, Mietus JE, Liu Y et al (1999) Exaggerated heart rate oscillations during two meditation techniques. *Int. J. Cardiol.* **70**(2): 101–107.

Price S (1993) *The Aromatherapy Workbook.* Thorsons, Wellingborough, UK.

Raghuraj P, Telles S (1997) Muscle power, dexterity skill and visual perception in community home girls trained in yoga or sports and in regular schoolgirls. *Indian J. Physiol. Pharmacol.* **41**(4): 409–415.

Raju PS, Prasad KV, Venkata RY et al (1997) Influence of intensive yoga training on physiological changes in six women: a case report. *J. Altern. Compleme. Med.* **3**(3): 291–295.

Rossi T, Melegari M, Bianchi A et al (1988) Sedative, anti-inflammatory and anti-diuretic effects induced in rats by essential oils of varieties of *Anthemis nobilis*: a comparative study. *Pharmacol. Res. Commun.* **200**(Suppl 5): 71–74.

Schaller KJ (1996) Tai Chi Chuan: an exercise option for older adults. *J. Gerontol. Nursing* **22**(10): 12–17.

Scheiber MD, Rebar RW (1999) Isoflavones and postmenopausal bone health: a viable alternative to estrogen therapy? *Menopause* **6**(3): 233–241.

Schmidt T, Wijga A, Von-zur-Muhlen A et al (1997) Changes in cardiovascular risk factors and hormones during a comprehensive residential three month kriya yoga training and vegetarian nutrition. *Physiol. Scand. Suppl.* **640**: 158–162.

Seidl MM, Stewart DE (1998) Alternative treatments for menopausal symptoms. A systematic review of scientific and lay literature. *Can. Family Phys.* **44**: 1299–1308.

Selvamurthy W, Sridharan K, Ray US et al (1998) A new physiological approach to essential hypertension. *Indian J. Physiol. Pharmacol.* **42**(2): 205–213.

Singer A, Wonnemann M, Muller WWE (1999) Hyperforin, a major antidepressant constituent of St John's wort, inhibits serotonin uptake by elevating free intracellular Na$^+$. *J. Pharmacol. Exp. Ther.* **290**(3): 1363–1368.

Southwell IA, Markham C, Mann C (1997) Skin irritancy of tea tree oil. *Essential Oil Res.* **9**: 47–52.

Stachenfeld NS, Maack GW, DiPietro L et al (1998) Regulation of blood volume during training in postmenopausal women. *Med. Sports Exerc.* **30**(1): 92–98.

Stephens FO (1999) The rising incidence of breast cancer in women and prostate cancer in men. Dietary influences: a possible preventive role for nature's sex hormone modifiers – the phytoestrogens. *Oncol. Rep.* **6**(4): 865–870.

Stone J (1999) Using complementary therapies in nursing: some ethical and legal considerations. *Complem. Ther. Nursing Midwif.* **5**: 46–50.

Stradling J, Roberts D, Wilson A, Lovelock F (1998) Controlled trial of hypnotherapy for weight loss in patients with obstructive sleep apnoea. *Int. J. Obes. Rel. Metab. Dis.* **22**(3): 278–281.

ter Riet G, Kleijnen J, Knipschild P (1990) Acupuncture and chronic pain: a criteria-based meta-analysis. *J. Clin. Epidemiol.* **43**(11): 1191.

UKCC (1992) *Code of Professional Conduct.* UKCC, London.

UKCC (1996) *Guidelines for Professional Practice.* UKCC, London.

Ulacia JCO, Paniagua RG, Luengo JM et al (1999) Models of intervention in menopause: proposal of a holistic or integral model. *Menopause* **6**(3): 264–272.

Vickers AJ, Fisher P, Smith C et al (1998) Homeopathic arnica 30× is ineffective for muscle soreness after long-distance running: a randomized double-blind placebo-controlled trial. *Clin. J. Pain* **14**(3): 227–231.

Wallis J (1994) Can osteopathy help relieve menopausal symptoms? *Prof. Nurse* **10**(2): 98.

Warenik-Szymankiewicz A, Meczekalski B, Obrebowska A (1997) Feminon N in the treatment of menopausal symptoms. *Ginekol. Pol* **68**(2): 89–93.

Whitten PL, Natfolin F (1998) Reproductive action of phytoestrogens. *Baillieres Clin. Endocrinol. Metab.* **12**(4): 667–690.

Williams LR, Stockley JK, Yan W, Home VN (1998) Essential oils with high antimicrobial activity for therapeutic use. *Int. J. Aromather.* **8**(4): 30–40.

Wolf SL, Barnhart HX, Kutner NG et al (1996) Reducing frailty and falls in older persons: an investigation of Tai Chi and computerized balance training. *J. Am. Geriatr. Soc.* **44**(5): 489–497.

Wolfson L, Whipple R, Derby C et al (1996) Balance and strength training in older adults: intervention gains and Tai Chi maintenance. *J. Am. Geriatr. Soc.* **44**(5): 498–506.

Wyon Y, Lindgren R, Lindeberg T, Hammar M (1995) Effects of acupuncture on climacteric vasomotor symptoms, quality of life and urinary excretion of neuropeptides among postmenopausal women. *Menopause* **2**: 3.

Yardley L, Furnham A (1999) Attitudes of medical and non-medical students towards orthodox and complementary therapies: is scientific evidence taken into account? *J. Altern. Compleme. Med.* **5**(3): 293–295.

Young DR, Appel LJ, Jee S, Miller ER (1999) The effects of aerobic exercise and Tai Chi on blood pressure in older people: results of a randomized trial. *J. Am. Geriatr. Soc.* **47**(3): 277–284.

Zarno V (1994) Candidiasis. *Int. J. Aromather.* **6**(2): 20–23.

9

Patient Support

It is acknowledged that HRT offers women relief from menopausal symptoms as well as conferring long-term benefits to many body systems. The media have widely publicized the risks associated with HRT use, but women often have a poor understanding of the potential benefits, other than those of symptom relief (Sinclair et al 1993).

So, do British women decline HRT because of known risks and expected side-effects, or are they simply unaware of the availability of HRT and therefore do not request it? In Scotland, a study showed that, of the 1100 women surveyed, many had experienced menopausal symptoms for over 6 months, yet 70% had not even considered HRT and nearly 80% had not discussed the matter with a doctor (Sinclair et al 1993). Most women want more information, not just about HRT, but also about the menopause itself (Draper & Roland 1990, Roberts 1991). Such information is surely most useful to a woman before the menopause, to prepare her for what is to come and allow her time to consider all the facts as they apply to her circumstances.

This chapter suggests ways of providing the information necessary for a woman to decide for herself whether HRT is appropriate.
Certainly some women will choose not to take HRT, but let us
ensure that their decision is based on accurate facts and not on
assumptions and myths; this, then, is truly an 'informed choice'. The
chapter also contains questions that are commonly asked by women
about HRT. Reading them will help to increase your awareness of
potential concerns and also broaden your knowledge of the subject.

DECISION-MAKING

Unlike may areas of medicine, the advice about whether to take
HRT is often not clearcut: it is appropriate for some women and not
for others. You cannot simply advise a woman that she would be
foolish to refuse HRT, as you might advise a diabetic who needs
insulin. With a condition such as diabetes, the facts are clearcut
and the consequences of not taking insulin profound. In the area of
HRT, you may need to spend a great deal of time discussing perceived risks and benefits as they apply to the individual woman
concerned.

We talk about helping a woman to make 'an informed choice'
about HRT, rather than simply telling her what to do. Sometimes it
can be hard to allow a woman to make her choice, which may not be
that which you would recommend. Yet women themselves expect to
do just that: to gather information and then to make their own
choice. There are well-known risks and benefits to taking HRT, but
the decision to take it is a complex one, requiring input and consideration from the individual as well as from the health professional. It
is not enough simply to advise a women: we must encourage her to
make a decision and then be prepared to help her carry it through.

Rothert et al (1990) have stated that there are three main factors
involved in making a decision about HRT:

◆ base rate risks
◆ perceived personal risk
◆ personal values.

In helping women decide about HRT, you can inform them of the base rate risk (e.g. of breast cancer) and assist them to assess their personal risk (e.g. of osteoporosis), while helping them to acknowledge their personal values (Rothert et al 1990).

Base rate risks relate to known facts, such as the incidence of osteoporosis or coronary heart disease after the menopause, the benefits of HRT and possible side-effects. These are common to all women and should be provided as background information to making a decision.

Perceived personal risk is influenced by actual experiences. Two women with identical medical backgrounds may perceive their personal risk in different ways. As health professionals we help to quantify the personal risk by making an assessment of risk factors, for example of heart disease or osteoporosis. Helping women to identify their risks enables them to make a suitable choice.

Personal values describe what is important to an individual woman. For example, some women are more concerned about breast cancer than heart disease. These women would be cautious about taking any medication that might increase their risk of breast disease, however small. Other women are more worried about strokes or heart attacks and are prepared to take a risk on the breast cancer issue. Some women consider the use of any hormones to be unnatural; others are not concerned about this issue. Personal values cannot be wrong and will vary from woman to woman. Any decision about HRT must be consistent with a woman's personal values if she is to persevere with the decision she had made.

SOURCES OF INFORMATION

Media

The subject of 'the change', and in particular HRT, is very popular with the press. Women's magazines, radio programmes and daily newspapers have all covered some aspect of the subject over the

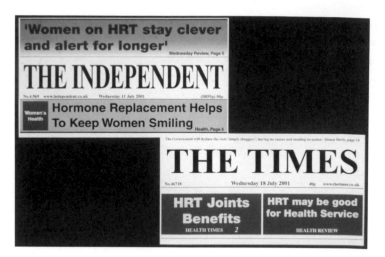

Figure 9.1 Headlines showing positive messages are often forgotten. Courtesy of the Medical Illustration Department, Northwick Park Hospital, Harrow.

past few years – some with greater accuracy than others (Fig. 9.1). Women themselves seem to find such articles very useful and many say that they are the main source of information after their general practitioner (GP).

Health professionals working in the field of menopause should try to keep up to date with media messages about HRT. Women may come to you to discuss such issues and it is helpful to be aware of the views expressed. Some articles are excellent and may be worth keeping as a resource, whereas others concentrate only on the perceived 'youth effects' of HRT, or highlight the frightening stories relating to HRT use.

Primary healthcare team

Most women who experience menopausal symptoms do not need referral to a hospital clinic. GPS can expertly treat and advise women, referring women to a specialist clinic only when necessary. However, some women express a general dissatisfaction with the advice received from their GP and some will travel many miles to be seen in a specialist clinic (Garnett et al 1991).

This may be because consultation times with GPs are too brief to cover adequately all aspects of the menopause and HRT. One survey revealed that the average GP consultation for menopause-related issues was 10 minutes, compared with 45 minutes with a specialist (Amarant Trust National Survey 1992). Some 80% of women questioned expressed dissatisfaction at this. Not surprisingly, women look elsewhere for accurate information. In response, some practices are recognizing the problem and seeking ways of providing information outside of general consultations with the GP. Practice nurses are becoming more involved in informing women about HRT and the menopause.

A survey of 800 practice nurses showed that 76% of practices were running a Well Woman Clinic, most providing some advice on the subject of menopause. In many practices, the role was shared equally between GPs and nurses, with a common pattern of care beginning with an assessment of a woman by the GP, who initiates therapy. After this the nurse counsels the woman on her chosen treatment and offers general lifestyle advice. However, 61% of the nurses surveyed identified a need for management protocols and 80% of respondents said they needed more training (Shine 1995). In a questionnaire survey of 144 practice nurses in northern England, only 27% of nurses stated that they were satisfied with their knowledge of HRT and the menopause (Roberts & Sibbald 2000). These issues need to be addressed before practice nurses can be expected to take on a greater role in menopause counselling.

There is no nationally recognized course (such as there is with family planning) dedicated to the subject of menopause and HRT, either for doctors or nurses. For doctors, training is usually through approved courses and study days as part of general post-basic education. Nurse education in menopause varies around the country, with some areas offering local courses whereas others have little in terms of training. Organizations such as the Amarant Trust, the National Osteoporosis Society, the British Menopause Society and Women's Health Concern have all organized study days for nurses and doctors on the subject of menopause and HRT. Some local specialist menopause clinics organize courses and study days.

Protocols

Defining a protocol of care (see Figs 9.2 & 9.3) will ensure that every woman receives the same high level of individual advice and assessment, whichever health professional they see. It also means that, within a team, each member knows what is expected and performs their role accordingly. It is important to define the care that can be taken on by the practice nurse and that which the doctor should perform. These roles and responsibilities will vary according to the training and competence of the nurse and the support and encouragement offered by the GP. Box 9.1 suggests how

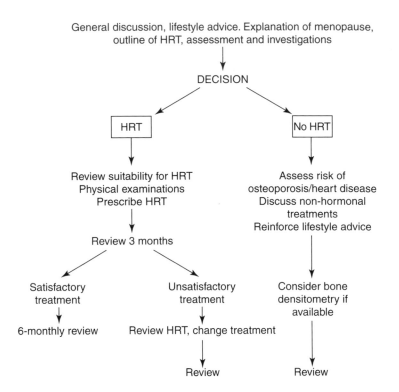

Figure 9.2 Suggested management plan for new patients.

Name ....

Hospital No.................................

Date of visit...............................

Visit No.......................

ON HRT? YES/NO

All answers are treated in the strictest confidence

The scoring system runs from 0–3 depending on the severity of your symptoms

Boxes under 0 – Not troubled at all
Boxes under 1 – Mildly troubled
Boxes under 2 – Moderately troubled
Boxes under 3 – Severely troubled

*Please clearly indicate your answer by placing an X against the appropriate box and please **do answer** all the questions. Thank you for your assistance; your answers will enable us to rapidly understand the severity of your problem and on subsequent visits, will help us identify the degree of success of the treatment.*

	QUESTIONS	0	1	2	3	Office use only
General problems:	Daytime sweats & flushes					
	Night-time sweats & flushes					
	Unable to sleep					
	Headaches					
	Tiredness					
	Loss of energy					
	General aches & pains					
	General itchiness					
	Formication (feeling of something crawling over you)					
Emotional problems:	Tearfulness					
	Depression					
	Feeling of unworthiness					
	Irritability					
	Anger					
	Bitterness					
	Panic attacks					
	+/– Palpitations					
	Aggression					
Bladder problems:	Daytime frequency					
	Urgency					
	Urge incontinence (leakage if you do not get there in time)					
	Stress incontinence (leakage if cough, sneeze or laugh)					
	Night-time frequency					
	Bed wetting					
Sexual problems:	Vaginal dryness/soreness					
	Vaginal itching					
	Soreness/pain with intercourse					
	Bleeding with intercourse					
	Loss of libido (sex drive)					
	Difficulty achieving orgasm					
Personality problems:	Loss of memory					
	Loss of concentration					
	Inability to cope					
	Feelings of personality disintegration					
Period problems:	Periods increasingly erratic					
	Periods much lighter					
	Periods much heavier					
	Irregular bleeding between periods					
	New bleed over 1 year after periods have stopped					

Figure 9.3 Menopause symptom assessment chart © Menopause Clinical and Research Unit, Northwick Park Hospital, Harrow.

Box 9.1 Suggested roles and responsibilities	
Nurse	**Doctor**
Initial identification of patients	Review suitability for HRT
Information and advice	Physical examination
Menopause	Secondary investigations
HRT	Initiate treatment
Lifestyle	6-Month check
Assessment for HRT	Change treatment if necessary
3-Month check	Regular checks, alternating
Regular checks, alternating with GP	with nurse
Be available to women for ongoing advice (telephone)	
Discussion of non-hormonal alternatives	
Identify problems and refer to GP	

responsibilities may be divided. There will usually be a degree of overlap where it is agreed that either the nurse or doctor is appropriate.

Providing information

Once it is recognized that a 10-minute consultation is insufficient for providing adequate information about menopause and therapy options, you can choose the method that is appropriate for your situation. Some doctors rely on the nurse to provide the basic information, whereas others will work together to help women come to a decision. The following may be helpful.

Group sessions. Some practice nurses have organized regular meetings to which women are invited to come to hear about the subject of menopause and HRT. During the session, general information about menopause and HRT is provided, outlining basic physiology, an introduction to HRT and some information about the long-term consequences of oestrogen deficiency. It is not designed to meet all individuals' needs, and women are invited to make a personal consultation with their doctor or practice nurse if appropriate. However, attendance at group sessions does mean that when a woman attends for her consultation she will already have the basic knowledge needed to ask relevant questions and perhaps make a decision for herself. For the nurse or GP, this is a valuable use of time, and for the women themselves it means that they probably have more time spent on information-giving and questions than would otherwise be the case.

Sometimes these meetings are open to any women who are interested, others are by invitation, targeting certain women, perhaps by age or medical history (e.g. hysterectomized women or those using corticosteroid therapy).

A disadvantage of this type of group is that some women may overwhelm the meeting and others may get a distorted view of HRT from any individuals who have not found a suitable type for themselves. Another drawback is that, for some women, group meetings can be very threatening, particularly if they consider the menopause to be a personal issue. The very people who need the information may not come at all. Other women will be very grateful for the opportunity to discuss the issue without feeling an obligation at least to try HRT if that seems to be what the nurse or doctor recommends. A group meeting can be suitably anonymous for those who want it to be! If you are in an area with a high population of a particular ethnic group, you may consider holding an information evening specifically for them, involving a community representative and translator if necessary, taking into account the needs of that particular ethnic group.

Some practices have put together a complete programme of meetings over about 6 weeks, covering issues such as:

◆ what is the menopause?
◆ lifestyle issues at mid life
◆ well woman care

- ◆ HRT
- ◆ osteoporosis
- ◆ heart disease
- ◆ sexuality and relationships
- ◆ alternative therapies.

These meetings may be organized in conjunction with several health professionals, including practice nurses, health visitors, family planning nurses, pharmacists, GPs and dieticians.

Support groups. Support groups differ from group information meetings in that support group members are encouraged to feel sufficiently comfortable to talk in a safe, supportive environment. There may be a health professional present, but the women themselves often lead or contribute to the meeting. It can be encouraging for a woman who is suffering symptoms to discover that what she is experiencing is not unusual. A woman can feel isolated, particularly if she is younger than average, and she may be unable to express her concerns to friends or family. Meeting women in a similar situation can be very useful.

Some suggestions for leading a support group are:

- ◆ Choose your venue, making it easily accessible, welcoming and comfortable.
- ◆ Introduce yourself and state the purpose of the group.
- ◆ Keep discussion going, asking leading questions and inviting people to contribute.
- ◆ Be prepared for a dominant group member, redirecting the discussion if necessary.
- ◆ Be aware of the time, finishing promptly.
- ◆ Review the group regularly.

Individual targeting. You may consider that it is most important to aim your information at those women who are known to have risk factors for osteoporosis or heart disease. If you have computerized records, you will be able to decide on certain risk factors and individually target women with those risks. Risk factors you may include would be:

◆ early menopause
◆ early hysterectomy
◆ prolonged use of corticosteroid therapy
◆ strong family history of heart disease
◆ women who have already experienced one fracture since the age of 40 years
◆ episodes of amenorrhoea in the past (unrelated to pregnancy)
◆ history of anorexia nervosa.

This method has the advantage of reaching those women who are most likely to benefit from HRT, and the information can be related specifically at the risk factors involved. Women who are invited may be more likely to attend than with an open invitation, but it is important to be sure that women are not frightened by the thought that they have been targeted as a possible candidate for a disease.

Literature. Having good-quality literature available (see Fig. 9.4) for women to take away means that women can read at their own

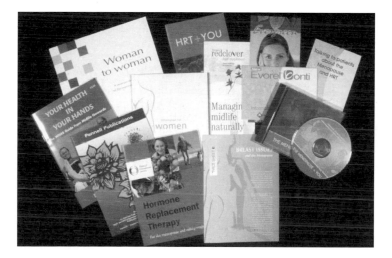

Figure 9.4 Various literature, courtesy of the Medical Illustration Department, Northwick Park Hospital, Harrow.

pace, share the information with their partners or friends, and return for discussion when they feel it is appropriate. Leaflets may be useful in that they are often provided free of charge to clinics and are unbiased towards any particular product, even though they are often provided by the pharmaceutical industry. However, they are usually strongly in favour of the use of HRT as opposed to trying alternative ways of relieving symptoms. They stress the benefits of long-term HRT, which can be useful for some women. Such literature should be used in addition to a full and frank discussion – not instead of it.

Literature can also be obtained from some of the health charities and organizations listed in the Appendix, but there may be a nominal charge for it. Some authorities have health promotion units which will act as a resource centre and give guidance about what may be available. Literature is available in languages other than English for those who need it.

Videos and books often go into much more detail about the issues involved, which is helpful to some women. The cost of such material, however, can make it difficult to provide in a clinic situation. It may be helpful to ask your local library to consider stocking books about the subject, which you could then suggest.

Dedicated clinic

When there was additional funding available to practices for running specific clinics, menopause clinics were just one of the many clinics being held that were dedicated to a specific disease or client group. Asthma clinics, hypertension clinics, weight-loss clinics, 'stop smoking' clinics, and so on, became the norm for practices large enough to warrant them and with the staff to run them. Whether or not one agreed with the way they were established or the financial arrangements behind them, there is no doubt that some people liked the idea that a clinic would be run by someone who was both interested and knowledgeable in the subject, with appointment times that reflected the consultations required and in a room or rooms that were conducive to the tests or investigations necessary (Roberts 1996).

Aims

In deciding to establish a clinic, consider what you hope to achieve. Do you simply wish to make information more widely available or do you hope to reach specific women who would not otherwise attend? Is your long-term aim to reduce fractures and cardiovascular incidents or do you hope to help symptomatic women in the short term? Considering such issues will help you to identify the best means to achieve these aims, in your situation. You will need to consider your own particular patient population: Will daytime appointments be useful or do most women work? Will women feel safe attending the clinic in the dark evenings? Do you have a particular ethnic group that you are hoping to inform – would you value an interpreter? Consider the literacy level of your likely group and tailor the literature accordingly.

If you decide to run a menopause clinic, you are implying to your patients that this is an issue that concerns you enough to try to improve the care that is given at this time. Women themselves seem to like clinics dedicated to issues such as menopause or family planning, but because they are not always cost effective, many practices cannot afford to run them. This does not mean, of course, that the treatment is any less effective when prescribed from a general clinic, or even that the staff are any less sympathetic, but it does occasionally mean that time is too limited to give all that is really needed.

Benefits of a dedicated clinic are:

◆ longer appointment times
◆ sympathetic and knowledgeable staff
◆ incorporates well-woman advice alongside specific menopause advice
◆ counselling, assessing and monitoring all done in same clinic.

Disadvantages of dedicated clinics are:

◆ appointment times are fixed
◆ patient loses her choice of doctor

- ◆ work can be repetitive for staff
- ◆ competing demands on staff time
- ◆ fragmentation of care by GPs.

Audit

Audit is simply a means of measuring standard of care. Audit can be as simple or as complex as you choose, depending on what you are trying to measure and over what period of time. One reason for audit is to ensure that standards of care are being maintained, even when a variety of health professionals is involved. Aims or goals can be set, a protocol established to meet those aims, and then an audit will help to measure the effectiveness of the activity. As a result of audit, you may choose to rethink your protocol in order to be more effective at reaching your stated goals or aims. An example is shown in Figure 9.5.

In relation to menopause and HRT in primary care settings, you may consider an audit of the following:

- ◆ number of hysterectomized women not on HRT
- ◆ why women in your practice stop HRT
- ◆ how many women in your practice have continued on HRT for more than 5 years
- ◆ number of women who have had both ovaries removed but are not on HRT.

Community pharmacists

Pharmacists have an important role to play in educating women about HRT and ensuring that they understand how to take their treatment, when prescribed. A woman may seek the advice of the community pharmacist about her HRT, particularly with regard to issues such as side-effects or practicalities of when or how to use the treatment. Therefore, it is important that the pharmacists have accurate information to hand, otherwise it can lead to more confusion on the part of the client. Practice nurses and GPs can help the local pharmacists by keeping them informed of any new regimens that are commonly prescribed, particularly if they are 'tailor-made'

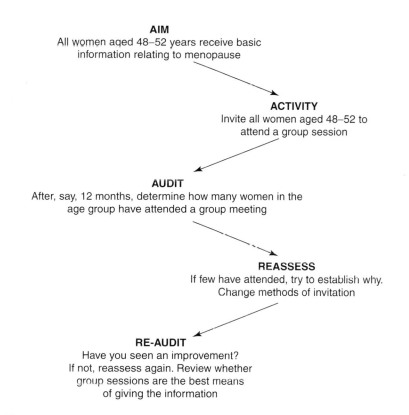

AIM
All women aged 48–52 years receive basic
information relating to menopause

ACTIVITY
Invite all women aged 48–52 to
attend a group session

AUDIT
After, say, 12 months, determine how many women in the
age group have attended a group meeting

REASSESS
If few have attended, try to establish why.
Change methods of invitation

RE-AUDIT
Have you seen an improvement?
If not, reassess again. Review whether
group sessions are the best means
of giving the information

Figure 9.5 Reassessing protocol following audit.

regimens. In turn, pharmacists can help GPs and nurses by being a resource about new products and treatments, and offering advice about prescribing problems.

QUESTIONS PATIENTS ASK*

Once you start to discuss with women about menopause and HRT, you will soon find that they turn to you for help and advice about their treatment. They may not have fully understood how to use the HRT, or they may be experiencing difficulties once they are on

*Some of these were first published in *Community Nurse* (Abernethy 1995).

it. It is helpful to encourage women to contact you if they do have anxieties or concerns, as many minor problems can easily be solved through a telephone conversation, saving the need for a further appointment. If women are unable to obtain help about a particular problem, they are more likely simply to stop treatment of their own accord. Women may also be returning to you for regular monitoring. It is important that they feel able to express any concerns and that you try to resolve any problems they may have. If women are able to ask questions, they will have more confidence in their HRT and also have a greater understanding of the treatment they have been prescribed.

Do I need HRT?

This is a difficult question to answer because the needs vary greatly between individuals. You should discuss a woman's symptoms and how much they are bothering her at present. What one woman might find intolerable, another will cope with more readily, depending on her lifestyle and work demands. It is also helpful to establish what the woman herself expects from HRT – is she realistic in considering the benefits? You should also discuss her risk of heart disease and osteoporosis, as this may be an influencing factor in her decision to take HRT. You can discuss her symptoms individually and consider how she could approach them from an alternative or complementary view.

After a frank discussion about her symptoms, risk of heart disease and osteoporosis, as well as a frank discussion about the side-effects and risks of HRT, you will be in a better position to help her decide whether to try HRT.

Do I need a blood test?

Women often believe that a blood test will help to determine whether they need HRT or not. However, most women do not need a blood test as actual levels of circulating oestrogen do not directly correlate to severity of symptoms. Follicle stimulating hormone (FSH) levels fluctuate widely during the perimenopause, even while symptoms may be quite severe. Measuring FSH levels may be useful in women who have had a hysterectomy, and are vital for the diagnosis of premature menopause, but in many other circumstances patient history alone is sufficient for a diagnosis.

Will HRT help all my symptoms?

If an adequate dose of HRT is taken, symptoms caused by oestrogen deficiency will gradually disappear. Problems arise when a woman experiences symptoms that arise around the time of the menopause but which may not be truly hormone related. This may include symptoms such as tiredness, irritability, loss of libido and headaches. While such symptoms may be caused by oestrogen deficiency, they may equally be caused by other influencing factors in a woman's life. It may be worth trying HRT, but you should advise a woman that HRT is not necessarily the answer.

What is the best form of HRT?

Women are becoming more aware of the different types of HRT – pills, patches, gels, nasal spray and implants – and may seek advice as to which one is the best. The answer is to choose a route with which the woman herself feels comfortable and to encourage her to persevere with this therapy for at least 3 months. Later, doses may need changing, progestogens may need adjusting, but ultimately the 'best' HRT is the one that suits the woman at that particular time. Both women themselves and health professionals need to be flexible enough to recognize that some treatments will suit some women more than others.

Aren't I just delaying the inevitable?

Taking HRT does not delay the menopause itself. It simply masks the fact that these hormonal changes are occurring. Women on HRT do not experience the menopause all over again when they stop HRT, although they may have a few symptoms if they do not stop HRT gradually. The menopause will occur whether or not HRT is taken; oestrogen simply makes the transition through the climacteric easier for some women.

How do I know the dose of HRT is right for me?

Women must feel confident that the HRT prescribed for them is not only effective but also safe. If a woman is taking HRT for symptom relief, the right dose is that which controls her symptoms adequately without too many side-effects. For those taking HRT for prevention of osteoporosis there is a standard dose of each preparation that is considered to be bone protective (see Ch. 3). For reassurance, bone densitometry may be necessary, particularly in women at a perceived high risk of fracture.

Can I safely take other medications alongside my HRT?

You can safely take other prescribed medications whilst using HRT, although you should advise your doctor that you are taking HRT. You can also take vitamins or dietary supplements if you wish. Some medications (e.g. antiepileptics) will affect the efficacy of HRT.

Can I get pregnant on HRT?

Women who are truly postmenopausal can be reassured that, even though they may see a return of bleeding, they are not fertile again. Women who start HRT while perimenopausal could theoretically get pregnant, so are advised to continue using a contraceptive method alongside their HRT (see Ch. 5). HRT alone should not be considered contraceptive.

Can I adjust the dose of HRT I take, according to how I am feeling?

Fluctuations of oestrogen often cause symptoms. The aim of HRT is to achieve a steady level of oestrogen circulating in the body, whilst maintaining a safe effect on the body. It is therefore unhelpful repeatedly to change the amount of HRT you take. However, you may find that the dose of oestrogen you require changes over the time that you take HRT. For example, you may need a higher dose when you start and a lower dose later on. You should discuss this with your doctor or practice nurse, who will help you to assess the dose you require.

Could HRT be causing my headaches, rather than relieving them?
Headaches may occur as a menopausal symptom, particularly in association with tiredness and poor sleep pattern. Headaches can also occur if the dose of oestrogen in HRT is not right for you. Some women experience headaches as a side-effect of progestogen in cyclical HRT. Headaches can also be caused by many other factors, such as stress, anxiety or poor eyesight. If you continue to suffer headaches whilst on HRT, it may be worth trying a different type or dose, while also trying to establish whether there is another cause for them.

Can I simply stop HRT without causing any harm?
It is quite safe simply to stop HRT at the end of a cycle. However, you may experience mild symptoms again, as your body gets used to a lower oestrogen level. It therefore makes sense to stop the oestrogen gradually over a 2–3-month period. You can do this by taking the oestrogen on alternate days, or by changing patches less frequently than usual. Meanwhile, if you have not had a hysterectomy, it is important that you continue taking the progestogen part of the regimen as normal until all oestrogen has been stopped. This may mean having the oestrogen and progestogen prescribed separately rather than in one pack for a short while. If you have had an implant, you may need to continue the progestogen for much longer, even if you are no longer having oestrogen implants (see Ch. 6).

I am going to have an operation. Do I need to stop my HRT?
There is usually no need to stop HRT before surgery. However, some surgeons and anaesthetists will advise that HRT is stopped up to 6 weeks before an operation because of the potential risk of thrombosis. This will depend on the type of surgery. You should check well in advance or you could risk having your operation

cancelled at the last moment. Surgery itself can be a risk factor for venous thrombosis; however, there are precautions that may be taken to reduce the risk of thrombosis, such as wearing elastic stockings or using medication to prevent clotting.

I have been taking HRT for 9 weeks, but it does not seem to be working – shall I try a different one?

You should try to persevere with a particular HRT for at least 3 months before deciding that it does not suit you. Some women take longer than others to 'settle' on to a therapy. If, after about 3 months on a particular HRT, you still feel that it is ineffective, return for further assessment. You may require an increase in dose or a change in the type of HRT.

I have been prescribed HRT, but when should I actually start it?

If you are still seeing periods, you should start your HRT near the beginning of a natural cycle, so that your bleeding remains regular in the early few months on HRT. If your periods have finished, you can start HRT as soon as you wish.

How soon can I expect to see an improvement in my symptoms?

Flushes and sweats often start to improve very quickly – even within 2–3 weeks of starting HRT. Other symptoms may take much longer to improve; some psychological symptoms may take months to improve. Most symptoms are improved by 6 months.

When will my bleed start and how long should it be?

If you are taking a cyclical form of HRT your bleed will come towards the end of the progestogen phase of treatment, or shortly afterwards (usually the end of the packet or the very beginning of the next). If it regularly starts much earlier than this you may need a change of dose of progestogen. Most women on cyclical HRT experience between 4 and 7 days of bleeding, although it can be much shorter than this. Women using a continuous oestrogen–progestogen regimen may experience irregular bleeding for several months, eventually settling to no bleeding at all in most cases. If you see a change in your regular bleeding pattern, you should seek advice.

After several years on cyclical HRT, my bleeds have now stopped altogether – does this matter?

A small proportion of women on cyclical HRT do not bleed at all, even though they are taking the progestogen regularly. When a woman has been on HRT for many years, the endometrium can become atrophic, so no bleeding occurs. This is considered satisfactory, although an ultrasonographic scan may be performed to ensure that the womb lining is not thickened. If it does appear thickened (usually greater than 4 mm), an endometrial biopsy may be performed to ensure that no unhealthy changes have occurred. This may be the time to consider changing to a 'period-free' regimen.

Can I delay my bleed so that the timing is more convenient, for example on holiday?

If you have been using HRT for some time, you can often change the timing of your bleed by adjusting the timing of the progestogen. It is best to do so gradually, over a couple of months before the one you wish to change, gradually delaying or bringing forward the progestogen so that the timing of the bleed changes. It should work, but you may see some occasional spotting instead of a regular bleed.

How do I change from monthly bleeds to a 'period-free' HRT?

Women who are at least 1 year past their last natural period or who are over 54 years of age may prefer to try a 'period-free' HRT. You should stop at the end of a packet and finish your withdrawal bleed. Then start the new treatment. There may be a settling-in phase of several months before all bleeding stops.

Does it matter if I take my HRT pills in the morning or at night?

For most women, it does not make any difference what time of day the tablets are taken. A few women experience mild nausea if they take tablets first thing in the morning, so prefer to take them later in the day or at night. It is important to try to take them at roughly the same time each day, whether morning or evening, simply to make it easier to remember.

What do I do if I miss a pill or a patch?

If you miss a pill, it is not worth trying to 'catch up' by taking two together next day. Simply leave the one you missed and continue with the regimen. If you miss a tablet during the progestogen phase, you may see some light bleeding a couple of days later. You should try not to miss too many pills because you may see a return of your symptoms within a short time. If you forget to change a patch, simply change it when you remember, then change it again on the day that it would normally be next due. It is most convenient if you always try to change your patch on the same day(s) of the week, as this makes it easier to remember.

Can I sunbathe or use a sunbed while wearing a patch?

It is advised that the patch should be covered or removed while using a sunbed. Ordinary sunbathing should not affect the patch. If you have slight allergy to a patch, sunbathing may make it worse.

Can I swim and shower while using a patch?

Newer patches are designed to stay on while you swim or shower. You may find that older style reservoir patches fall off in a prolonged hot bath. These patches can be dried and reapplied after the bath if necessary, although this may make them less effective.

Does it matter where I put the patch or gel?

Patches should be applied below the waistline, usually to the buttock or abdomen. Gel should be applied to the upper arms or inner thigh area. It is common sense to avoid using the same area of skin all the time when changing your patches: change the site regularly and avoid applying a patch or gel to an area of broken skin.

Can I use natural progesterone cream instead of conventional progestogen with my HRT?

In theory you might, provided you could be sure of the dose and absorption you were getting. At present, these data are not available. This means that you are at risk of experiencing endometrial hyperplasia (build-up of the womb lining), a potentially harmful condition. Until more studies are available to establish its safety when used in this way, this is not recommended.

What do you mean by a 'healthy diet'?

The media would have us believe that a healthy diet is simply one that keeps us looking good. General recommendations for a healthy diet are wider than that, and include:

◆ reducing total fat intake
◆ reducing salt intake
◆ reducing sugar intake
◆ increased fibre, in the form of fruit and vegetables
◆ increased intake of starches and cereals.

For women, the importance of adequate calcium should be remembered. Calcium is found most easily in dairy products, but is also in green vegetables, sardines, skimmed milk powder and some fortified drinks such as orange juice or soya milk

CONCLUSION

Some would argue that all women from the age of 45 years upwards should receive information about the menopause even if they do not actually ask for it. This may simply mean providing literature in the waiting room, or raising the subject when they are in the surgery for something else. The most appropriate time may be when the woman attends for her regular cervical smear test. A brief comment or question can ensure that the woman knows that discussion is invited if and when she wishes. The woman is then free to raise the issue again, or simply to leave it at this time. Some women may not realize that help is available, or may be too embarrassed to raise the issue specifically. All nurses should be providing information to women about menopause, whether it is ward nurses, family planning nurses, health visitors, occupational health nurses or others. In some situations it is the nurse who is likely to be more available to give advice, and it is vital that such opportunities are taken.

It is only as women feel able to ask the necessary questions and to have an open, frank discussion that they can make a decision that is right for them. In order to do this, they need information not just about menopause and what it is, or HRT, but also about other health issues, lifestyle and non-hormonal therapies, as well as an understanding of the changes that occur in a woman's body at this time.

REFERENCES

Abernethy K (1995) Patients' top 10 HRT questions. *Community Nurse* 2: 38–39.
Amarant Trust (1992) *Amarant Trust National Survey*. Amarant Trust, London.
Draper J, Roland M (1990) Perimenopausal women's views on taking HRT to prevent osteoporosis. *Br. Med. J.* 300: 786–788.
Garnett T, Mitchell A, Studd J (1991) Patterns of referral to a menopause clinic. *J. R. Soc. Med.* 84: 128.
Roberts PJ (1991) The menopause and HRT – views of women in general practice receiving HRT. *Br. J. Gen. Pract.* 41: 421–424.
Roberts PJ (1996) Comparison of care between a general practice clinic and general surgeries: the views of women using HRT. *J. Br. Menopause Soc.* 2: 1.

Roberts PJ, Sibbald E (2000) Menopausal health care provision: the views of GPs and practice nurses. *J. Br. Menopause Soc.* **6**: 154–158.

Rothert M, Rovner D, Holmes M et al (1990) Women's use of information regarding HRT. *Res. Nurs. Health* **13**: 355–366.

Shine U (1995) The true facts on HRT. *Practice Nurse* 1 December: 528–529.

Sinclair HK, Bond CM, Taylor RJ (1993) HRT: a study of women's knowledge and attitudes. *Br. J. Gen. Pract.* **43**: 365–370.

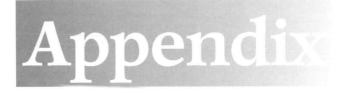

Resources

Aimed at the non-medical reader

Is it me or is it hot in here?, by Jenni Murray. Vermillion 2001

The menopause, HRT and you, by Caroline Hawkridge. Penguin 1999

Menopause – a practical self help guide for women, by Raewyn Mackenzie. Sheldon Press 1994

Understanding HRT and the menopause, by Robert C Wilson. Which? Books 1999

Hormone replacement therapy, by Miriam Stoppard. Dorling Kindersley 1999

The phyto factor, by Maryon Stewart. Vermillion 1998

Beat the menopause without HRT, by Maryon Stewart. Headline Book Publishing 1995

The silent passage, by Gail Sheehy. Harper Collins 1993

Aimed at health professionals

Hormone replacement therapy: a guide for primary care, edited by Sally Hope, Margaret Rees and Janet Brockie. Oxford University Press 1999.

Premature menopause – a multidisciplinary approach, edited by Myra Hunter and Dani Singer. Whurr Publishers 2000

Osteoporosis, by John A Kanis. Blackwell Science 1995

The Sheffield protocol for the management of the menopause and the prevention and treatment of osteoporosis, edited by Sue Lee. Sheffield 2000

The vital meridian, by A Bensouusan. Churchill Livingstone 1991

The nurse's handbook of complementary therapies, 2nd edn, by Denise Rankin-Box. Churchill Livingstone 2000

Essential oil safety: a guide for health professionals, by R Tisserand and T Balacs. Churchill Livingstone 1995

More than an old age problem: understanding osteoporosis. Educational video for nurses: Nursing Times Changing Practice series, Clinical Study Unit 15. Healthcare Productions 2000

Useful addresses

British Menopause Society
36 West Street
Marlow
Bucks
SL7 2NB
www.the-bms.org

Multidisciplinary professional organization for health professionals working in the field of menopause. At present the BMS does not have facilities for enquiries from the lay public.

National Osteoporosis Society
Camerton
Bath
BA2 0PJ
www.nos.org.uk

Provides excellent literature for both lay and health professionals at reasonable cost, on many issues relating to osteoporosis. Helpline available.

Women's Health
52–54 Featherstone Street
London EC1Y 8RT

Information available for lay women on many health-related issues.

The Amarant Trust
Sycamore House
5 Sycamore Street
London EC1Y OSR
Helpline: 01923 413000 (Mon–Fri 11 am to 6 pm)

Information available about menopause-related issues, mainly for lay women.

Family Planning Association
2–12 Pentonville Road
London N1 9FP
Helpline: 020 7837 4044 (contraceptive issues)

For information on any issue relating to reproductive and sexual health, for both lay and health professionals. Helpline available for issues relating to contraception only.

Women's Nutritional Advisory Service (WNAS)
PO Box 268
Lewes
East Sussex
BN7 2QN
www.wnas.org.uk

Offers specific dietary, nutritional and exercise advice for women with premenstrual syndrome or going through the menopause.

Women's Health Concern
PO Box 2126
Marlow
Bucks
SL7 2NB
Helpline: 01628 483612

Literature available on all aspects of women's health.

Relate
Head Office
Little Church Street
Rugby
CV21 3AP

The Pennell Initiative for Women's Health
Health Services Management Unit
University of Manchester
Devonshire House, Precinct Centre
Oxford Road
Manchester M13 9PL
Tel: 0800 550 220 for the Report
www. pennellwomenshealth.org

An organization dedicated to promoting and coordinating research into older women's health.

Daisy Network
PO Box 392
High Wycombe
Bucks
HP15 7SH

Premature menopause support and information.

British Homeopathic Association
15 Clerkenwell Close
London EC1R OAA
www.trusthomeopathy.org

British Herbal Medicine Association
PO Box 304
Bournemouth
Dorset
BH7 6JX

Complementary Therapies in Nursing, Special Interest Group
Royal College of Nursing
20 Cavendish Square
London W1M 0AB

Register of Qualified Aromatherapists
54a Gloucester Ave
London NW1 8JD

British Acupuncture Council
63 Jedda Road
London W12 9HQ
Info@acupuncture-org.uk

Foundation for Integrated Medicine
International House
59 Compton Road
London N1 2YT

Natural Progesterone Information Service
PO Box 24
Buxton
Derbyshire
SK17 9FB

Information packs on natural progesterone.

Index

Note: abbreviations used in the index are CAM = complementary and alternative medicine; HRT = hormone replacement therapy; SERM = selective (O) estrogen receptor modulator. Page numbers in **bold** refer to tables and boxes; page numbers in *italics* refer to figures.